The Optimized Woman

Using your menstrual cycle
to achieve success
and fulfillment

First published by O Books, 2009
O Books is an imprint of John Hunt Publishing Ltd., The Bothy, Deershot Lodge, Park Lane, Ropley,
Hants, SO24 0BE, UK
office1@o-books.net
www.o-books.net

Distribution in:

UK and Europe
Orca Book Services
orders@orcabookservices.co.uk
Tel: 01202 665432 Fax: 01202 666219
Int. code (44)

USA and Canada
NBN
custserv@nbnbooks.com
Tel: 1 800 462 6420 Fax: 1 800 338 4550

Australia and New Zealand
Brumby Books
sales@brumbybooks.com.au
Tel: 61 3 9761 5535 Fax: 61 3 9761 7095

Far East (offices in Singapore, Thailand,
Hong Kong, Taiwan)
Pansing Distribution Pte Ltd
kemal@pansing.com
Tel: 65 6319 9939 Fax: 65 6462 5761

South Africa
Alternative Books
altbook@peterhyde.co.za
Tel: 021 555 4027 Fax: 021 447 1430

Text copyright Miranda Gray 2008

Design: Stuart Davies

ISBN: 978 1 84694 198 6

A CIP catalogue record for this book is available
from the British Library.

Printed and bound by CPI Group (UK) Ltd, Croydon, CR0 4YY

O Books operates a distinctive and ethical publishing philosophy in
all areas of its business, from its global network of authors to
production and worldwide distribution.
This book is produced on FSC certified stock, within ISO14001
standards. The printer plants sufficient trees each year through
the Woodland Trust to absorb the level of emitted carbon in
its production.

The
Optimized
Woman

Using your menstrual cycle
to achieve success
and fulfillment

Miranda Gray

BOOKS

Winchester, UK
Washington, USA

CONTENTS

Acknowledgements

To my husband who continuously supports me in all my numerous creative projects.

To everyone who I have met both face to face and online who has contributed and supported this title. I feel honored at having met so many amazing women and appreciate your on-going input and help.

Preface

You simply have to look along the shelves in any bookstore to see the popularity of personal development, life-coaching and business-coaching subjects. And of course there are numerous courses and workshops to help you to transform yourself, your life and your career with goal setting, action plans and motivational schemes. So why do we need a new book on changing our lives? Because the books currently on the market are not specifically designed for women and don't take into account what makes them different to men!

We readily buy new self-help books to change our lives. We commit to the method, apply the techniques to our thought processes and activities, read the motivational statements, and then find that two or three weeks later we have lost that commitment and motivation, and the dream of success has gone.

So why don't these personal development systems work well for women? Because **women have something which men haven't got** – and these schemes fail to take this one important factor into account!

The Optimized Woman Daily Plan is a 28-day guide specifically designed to help women become aware of their **Optimum Times** and associated abilities, to apply them to create fulfillment and self-motivation, and to achieve the success and goals they want in their lives.

By taking action at the right time and using peak time abilities and talents when they arise, we are able to work with our natural motivation, creativity and insight to make the dramatic changes in our development and work lives that we really want.

The concept in this book is out-of-the-box; it is a new, unique approach that will radically change the way you think about yourself and how you live your life. Try the plan for 28 days and discover for yourself your own unique talents and skills and how to practically apply them to everyday situations and work projects and to the achievement of long-term goals. This book will change your self-perception, build your self-confidence, and help you to experience the vibrant, creative, successful woman that you truly are.

You will be amazed that this is the one self-development method that you can apply month after month without losing the commitment and motivation to achieve your dreams, and bring fulfillment and success.

Miranda Gray

"We all know the saying that if we want to change the world we must first change ourselves. But what if we change during the month; does that mean the world changes too? Yes."
Miranda Gray.

Chapter 1

Why 28 days?

What do women have that men don't?

What if I told you that you had a tremendous power available to you? What if I told you that it would empower you to go beyond your everyday expectations, bring focus and logical reasoning, create better relationships, enhance your problem solving ability, offer creative insight and blue-sky thinking, and finally, create deep insight and understanding?

What if I told you that you are not using the one greatest power source that you have at this moment which could make you more successful at work and in your life? Would you be interested? Of course you would!

And then, what if I said that the answer to 'What do women have and men don't?' is the menstrual cycle.

Bet you weren't expecting this!

> **The menstrual cycle is a huge unrealized personal and work asset.**

Generally the menstrual cycle is seen as an inconvenience rather than an advantage, and the worlds of business, work and personal development have completely ignored a fundamental truth about women: that our abilities change throughout the month.

Unlike men, we have a cycle of mental, physical and emotional changes which impacts the way we think, feel and behave. We have within our cycles a natural, in-built life-coaching model

1

with its own Optimum Times for planning, consolidating, taking action, creative thinking, reviewing and cutting loose.

Where other life transformation and goal achievement approaches go wrong is to force women into a linear structure with unrealistic expectations about the consistency of our mental and emotional approaches and perspectives. This limits us from reaching our full potential in a much wider and diverse range of abilities during our Optimum Times.

With current self-development techniques we are

"I found Miranda Gray's 28 day program to be very self empowering as a woman in the work place. It has allowed me to maximize my peak times and strengths throughout my cycle and to be a little more forgiving of those times when I didn't feel quite so energized and productive. I would recommend this program to any woman." Tess, Human Resources, Canada.

forced into a masculine way of thinking, creating the seeds of failure before we even start towards our goals. And in the business world, rigid working structures ignore our cyclic nature, losing businesses the best creative resource they may have – us!

When we do work in awareness of our abilities and talents as they occur during the month, we can become exceptionally productive and perceptive members of a working team and experience levels of achievement and personal fulfillment beyond our expectations, in our personal and work life.

In a world where every business needs an edge to keep ahead, tapping into the vast resource of abilities women offer could provide the necessary inspired leaps to stay one step ahead of competitors.

What are our 'Optimum Times' and how can we use them?

The monthly cycle consists of four Optimum Times. These are days when we experience specific heightened mental abilities, emotional qualities, intuitive awareness and physical aptitudes. On these days we have a unique opportunity to use our heightened abilities in a

> It is generally easier to concentrate on work and be more positive during my Dynamic and Expressive phases. I have more energy and can get a lot done.
>
> Barbara, Teacher, UK.

positive and dynamic way to reach our full potential. By becoming aware of our Optimum Times and the types of heightened abilities they contain for us, and by practically applying these abilities to our lives when they arise, we can not only discover new talents and achieve more, but finally live a life true to our female nature and excel at being ourselves.

Although some generalizations have had to be made for the purposes of this book, including the number of days in the plan, the 28-day plan will help guide you in discovering your own unique personal Optimum Times and abilities, regardless of how regular or how long you cycle is. The Optimized Woman Daily Plan can be used by women with either a natural or a medically managed cycle (for more information see *Chapter 8*).

Throughout the month most women experience a number of distinct phases. I have called these phases the *Dynamic phase*, the *Expressive phase*, the *Creative phase* and the *Reflective phase*.

> **The Optimized Woman Daily Plan is a guide to discovering your own unique Optimum Times and heightened personal abilities.**

3

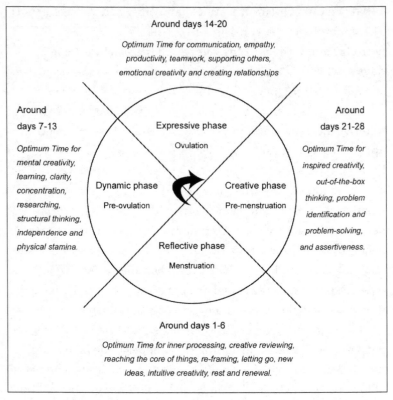

Around days 14-20

*Optimum Time for communication, empathy,
productivity, teamwork, supporting others,
emotional creativity and creating relationships*

Around
days 7-13

*Optimum Time for
mental creativity,
learning, clarity,
concentration,
researching,
structural thinking,
independence and
physical stamina.*

Expressive phase

Ovulation

Dynamic phase
Pre-ovulation

Creative phase
Pre-menstruation

Reflective phase

Menstruation

Around
days 21-28

*Optimum Time for
inspired creativity,
out-of-the-box
thinking, problem
identification and
problem-solving,
and assertiveness.*

Around days 1-6

*Optimum Time for inner processing, creative reviewing,
reaching the core of things, re-framing, letting go, new
ideas, intuitive creativity, rest and renewal.*

Figure 1 The cycle phases and Optimum Times

1. The **Dynamic phase**

This occurs after menstruation and before ovulation. It can be the Optimum Time for mental focus, concentration, learning, researching, structural thinking, independence and physical stamina.

2. The **Expressive phase**

This occurs around the time of ovulation, and can be the Optimum Time for communication, empathy, productivity, teamwork, supporting others, and creating inter-dependent relationships.

3. The **Creative phase**

More commonly known as the pre-menstrual phase, this can be the Optimum Time for creativity, inspiration, out-of-the-box thinking, problem identification and problem-solving, and assertiveness.

4. The **Reflective phase**

This is the menstrual phase itself, which can be the Optimum Time for inner processing, creative reviewing, reaching the core of things, re-framing, letting go, new ideas, rest and renewal.

Most of us try to override this natural cycle of abilities to fit into the structure of the modern world. Without knowledge of our Optimum Times we can often perceive our abilities and ourselves as inconsistent and unreliable, a view that may be shared by partners, bosses and co-workers.

We compensate by working extra hard, producing work which is not to our highest potential, taking stimulants to force our thinking and our bodies into 'the way it should be', and feeling unfulfilled because our life is a constant struggle to fit into a structure which does not fit us. It's a case of a round peg being hammered into a square hole.

The natural monthly life-coach

When we work within our natural cycle of Optimum Times, we also automatically have the skills we need to create success in both personal and business goals.

Most life-coaching methods suggest:

1. Setting a goal then researching and planning incremental steps towards it.

The abilities of the *Dynamic* phase of a cycle are ideal to apply to these tasks. These can include heightened mental focus and structural thinking.

2. Taking action and building relationships to help us achieve the goal.

5

The abilities of enhanced communication skills, confidence, productivity and sociability attached to the *Expressive* phase of a cycle can be used in networking and creating the necessary backing and support for our goals.

3.Using your creativity to actively solve problems and create a clear direction.

The cycle's *Creative* phase can be a potential powerhouse of inspiration and new ideas. Its heightened intolerance of the superfluous creates a clear focus for our goal.

4.Reviewing progress so far.

The tendency towards inner reflection and review in the *Reflective* phase of a cycle makes it an ideal time to review situations and goal progress.

Within one monthly cycle we naturally have all the abilities we need to become our own life-coach and to create and support the short and long term changes and successes we want to make in our lives!

> **Within the menstrual cycle we have a natural process of life-coaching.**

Actively using our Optimum Times

When we don't take the cycle into account we can take actions incompatible with our Optimum Time abilities. We may start new projects in a phase which is totally unsuitable, such as the Reflective phase, rather than in an Optimum Time which has the mental, emotional and physical abilities to enhance what we wish to achieve – in this case, the *Dynamic* phase.

Have you ever started a new diet or fitness regime and broken it within a couple of days? The chances are you started it in the *Creative* or *Reflective* phases.

We also tend to hold unrealistic expectations of having

constant abilities, which increases our levels of frustration and stress when we don't perform in accordance with these expectations.

In the *Expressive* phase, when our natural abilities are those of building and supporting productive relationships, it's unrealistic to continue to expect the high levels of mental focus and concentration of the *Dynamic* phase.

To reach our full potential we need to understand our Optimum Times and to actively use them in practical ways. The immediate response by women to this idea is often:

'You've got to be kidding, it's not like I can change my life / job / boss / the world to suit my cycle!'

This is perfectly understandable and true. We can't yet organize the world to suit our Optimum Times, but we can use awareness and where possible the practical application of our heightened cyclic abilities to create chances to get the best out of ourselves. This gives us the opportunity to shine at work, run successful projects and create the work-life balance we want.

> **Although the working world does not support the flexible abilities of women, we can actively use awareness of our Optimum Times to make the best use of our abilities to excel at work and create the success and life experience we want.**

The Optimized Woman Daily Plan is specifically designed to help you become aware of your Optimum Times and to actively use those times to reach your full potential for achieving your goals.

It's important to remember that we are talking about *Optimum Times*; this doesn't mean that you can't do work or tasks at any other time throughout the month, it simply means that if you match the task to the time you will shine. You may also surprise yourself with the new talents and abilities you discover.

> **If you match the task to the time you will shine.**

Who is the Optimized Woman Daily Plan for?

The Optimized Woman Daily Plan is designed for any woman who wants to discover the true depth of her abilities and how she can practically apply them to create the life she wants. The plan includes daily actions which target three main areas of life:

1. **Self-development:** consisting of actions for confidence, self-esteem, creativity, relationships, lifestyle, self-acceptance, exploring what it means to be you, and using the Optimum Times to enhance your sense of well-being.
2. **Goal achievement:** consisting of actions to identify your true goals, when and what steps to take, how to build motivation, and how to use your Optimum Times to provide the necessary support to achieve your goals and dreams.
3. **Work enhancement:** consisting of actions which include using your full potential, identifying the right work for you, working more effectively, and exploring the Optimum Time to do tasks and make decisions.

The plan can be used by any woman who experiences a pattern of changes related to her hormonal cycle, including medically managed cycles, ie. using hormonal contraception, as well as women who experience irregular cycles including the menopause. If you have an erratic cycle, or if it lasts longer or less than the 28 days outlined in the plan (and we all experience months like that), the plan is adaptable and designed to give you the ideas and inspiration to create your own unique plan from your personal experiences.

How did the Optimized Woman Daily Plan develop?

In the 1990s I wrote a book called *Red Moon – Understanding and Using the Gifts of the Menstrual Cycle*. Based on women's experiences of their menstrual cycles, I suggested an approach to the cycle which reflected its effects on women's creativity, mental processes, spirituality, sexuality, emotional healing and well-being.

The initial inspiration for the book came from my awareness of the effect my own cycle had on my work as self-employed illustrator, both creatively and on my business skills. Since the publication of *Red Moon* I have given workshops and talks in Europe and North America, and the main question I have heard again and again is 'What's the point of the menstrual cycle if I have had my children or don't want children yet?'

It has taken me over ten years of being the creative director of a multimedia development company and an enthusiastic practitioner and facilitator of self-development techniques to be able to answer this question in a way which is applicable to the everyday working environment and to life-coaching methods. The Optimized Woman Daily Plan is the answer.

Every woman's experience of her abilities and Optimum Times will be different and this book uses examples from my own experiences and those of other women to give ideas on what to look for and what to try. Our cycles offer us the keys to a female style empowerment to get ahead in the masculine world, and perhaps this book will inspire the first business or organization to allow women to actively work with this resource!.

The menstrual cycle has always been a part of society and culture and now it's back, and this time it's armed and dangerous!

> **By using the plan you will come to see your cycle as a practical resource for development and achievement.**

In the following chapters I will show you how you can use the four Optimum Times practically, in everyday life, at work, and to aid you in creating and achieving your goals. I will also introduce you to the plan and show you how to make it work for you.

Summary:

- The menstrual cycle is an untapped, potent source of invaluable abilities which can be actively used to enhance our lives and careers and to help us achieve the goals we desire.
- Our cycles can be divided into four phases which contain specific types of abilities and perceptions. These phases are the *Dynamic, Expressive, Creative* and *Reflective* phases. Our monthly cycle consists of a repeating pattern of heightened abilities.
- Each phase is an Optimum Time for particular abilities and actions. By utilizing these abilities within their Optimum Times we are able to create better results than we would achieve in other phases.
- The menstrual cycle has a natural life-coaching structure inherent within it. We can use our cycles to support our goals through planning, action, networking, creative thought, and review.
- The Optimized Woman Daily Plan will help you to recognize your natural abilities during the month and give you practical ideas on how you can use them to your advantage. It will also help you to plan actions in tune with your phases at work, and show you how to use the life-coaching aspect of your cycle.

- The plan can be used by any woman with a hormonal cycle, whether natural or medically managed. The plan is flexible enough to include irregular and erratic cycles of more or less than 28 days.
- Your cycle is a practical resource for personal, career and life development and achievement.

> "I wish I had had this information years ago.
>
> Understanding that there is more to the menstrual cycle means that I can now work with it rather than fight it. I've started the plan and I'm already planning out my month ahead." Amanda, Therapist, Australia.

Chapter 2

How to use this book

I know there will be many readers who will want to get started on the Optimized Woman Daily Plan straight away, and there's no reason you can't turn directly to the plan in *Chapter 9*. I have however found when working with women on the ideas in the plan that understanding a little more about the changes associated with each Optimum Time and being given additional examples of practical ways of using the associated abilities helped them to recognize what to look for as they experienced their cycles. Also, there are a number of key approaches to the plan which can help it to become more readily an active part of everyday life.

The following section, *The Keys to 28-day success*, provides guidelines on the best approach for working with The Optimized Woman Daily Plan, and *Chapter 3: Getting to know your phases* provides a general overview of the cycle and how it works.

When we understand what is happening to us within our cycles, it becomes easier to accept our changes, to enjoy them and to find fun and unique ways of using them in our everyday lives. The chapters on each of the four phases explore each phase in detail, looking at the mental, emotional and physical changes we can experience, and provide practical strategies on using the abilities available in these Optimum Times. They also cover how to avoid expectations and actions which will clash with the phase - it always helps to know what not to do as well as what to do.

It always helps to know what not to do as well as what to do!

The Optimized Woman Daily Plan acts as an initial guide to help you to discover your own Optimum Time abilities and how you can use them to your best advantage. You may want to use the plan as it is, or after trying it for a cycle you may want to create your own plan tailored to fit your unique cycle. To help you do this, *Chapter 10: Done the Plan, So what's next?* shows you how to create a more in-depth record of your cyclic abilities using a *Cycle Dial*. Your Cycle Dial can become your own unique power map for getting the best from your cycle and the ultimate guide to unlocking your potential for success, goal achievement and happiness.

The keys to 28-day success

There are five key approaches we need to apply to our cycle to use our heightened abilities in their Optimum Times in a way which is not only applicable to everyday life but actually works. The Key approaches are:

Key 1: Awareness
Key 2: Planning
Key 3: Trust
Key 4: Action
Key 5: Flexibility

Key 1: Awareness

Awareness is the most important key to releasing our potential talents and working with the heightened abilities of our cycles, and it is the underlying factor in all the other keys.

"A very interesting month. It has made me aware that some physical, mental and emotional abilities are linked to a cycle." Melanie, Teacher, UK

13

To fulfill our full potential and perhaps discover new talents we need to be consciously aware of the changes in our bodies, mental aptitude and emotional qualities as we journey through each month.

Without noticing what we find easy or difficult and relating it to our cycle, we won't know when our abilities are at their best, and will miss out on the powerful resources these Optimum Times offer. We may experience failing at projects, goals and tasks simply because we are taking the wrong actions at the wrong time.

Being self-aware not only helps us to achieve more and do better but it also builds self-confidence and self-esteem. It helps us to discover the real 'me' and to understand that being 'inconsistent' is not a negative aspect of being female but is instead life-enhancing and empowering.

Key 2: Planning

Awareness of our Optimum Times through use of the plan for a number of months brings the solid realization that our heightened abilities are cyclic; that they occur around the same time each month.

This wonderful revelation empowers us to plan in advance how to use our heightened abilities to our best advantage in the following month. We can dynamically plan to use them to benefit everyday tasks, to produce better results at work, or we can apply them to our goals and dreams to enhance our progress. We can set goals for the month ahead, but unlike with traditional life-coaching we set our goal actions in tune with our cycle.

> **The plan alongside our diary becomes a powerful tool to achieve success and personal fulfillment.**

Planning ahead enables us to set everything up in advance so we have all the necessary information or component parts in the right place at the right time for us to complete the task at hand quickly and efficiently. Our heightened abilities therefore go into the task rather than being wasted in trying to organize everything necessary.

Planning does however depend on trust. We have to trust that if we leave a job until the following week's expected heightened abilities, they will appear. It can be a real challenge when the Optimum Time for a task begins just before its deadline.

Key 3: Trust

One of the most difficult things when we start to work with our Optimum Times is to trust that the 'magical' abilities will come. Conversely, we also have to realize that this level of heightened ability does not stay around forever, so we have to trust that we can work effectively with our abilities as they change.

It takes awareness, and the experience of putting that awareness into plans and actions, for us to be able to trust the process we go through each month. The reward for that trust is often a 'wow' factor – perhaps discovering a new ability or achieving something beyond our expectations.

Trust means, where possible, that we leave a task until its Optimum Time. This can be a real challenge, especially in pressurized circumstances where the impression of leaving a task until later can suggest that the task has 'low priority'. In fact we are giving it our highest priority by leaving it until our Optimum Time. When we trust in our abilities, our co-workers will trust in them too, because we produce good work and deliver on time. We simply need to be a little more assertive about the timescales for a job.

As I run my own business, you may think that it's easy for me as I can organize my own working life. Well, yes and no. Yes, it is a little easier for me to be a bit more flexible with the way I work, but I still have to meet deadlines set by others, whether they are clients, suppliers, or co-workers. I still have to go to meetings, write reports, and communicate with the world, all at times which are not optimum for those tasks. Where possible I try to arrange tasks to fit in with my heightened abilities, but it's not always possible. It doesn't mean that I can't do the work at any other time of the month, it just means that I am simply not working on it at my full potential.

We have to trust our Optimum Times enough to say to ourselves; 'Yes, I know it's urgent but my optimum skills are due next week. I will leave it until then but will keep aware just in case the skills appear early. If you remember, the last time I left a task until the Optimum Time I achieved so much more in much less time.'

The more we work with our Optimum Times, the more we will trust our ability to achieve goals and create successes and the more the people around us will trust the unique way we handle tasks.

Key 4: Action

The only way we are going to trust our cyclic abilities is to take the right action during the right Optimum Time. We have to put the concept into action if we are to experience the unique effects our Optimum Times have for us.

The plan is designed to give you ideas and suggestions of daily actions for 28 days in three specific areas of your life. These areas are *self-development, goal achievement* and *work enhancement.*

You can choose the daily actions for one specific area and spend a month trying them out, or you can select one or more of the actions to try each day.

It's important to try to apply our Optimum Time abilities practically, even if it's on something small. For example, we may experience a higher than usual level of mental concentration and focus during our *Dynamic* phase, so why not use this time to do our accounts and check through financial arrangements and purchases, perhaps looking for better deals or prices? In this phase we're more able to process complex information, to spot errors, do the math, and understand the small print. It will also take less time to go through, and we're less likely to get bored by the whole thing.

If we don't take action during our Optimum Times, we'll lose the opportunity to experience a higher level of abilities (which will generate increased trust in our skills), and we will also waste a valuable opportunity to complete a task quickly and easily.

> **Potential talents will become actual skills.**

Key 5: Flexibility

Flexibility is necessary because we don't run like clockwork. The total length of the cycle can alter and it can become more regular or irregular, varying the length of time for each Optimum Time. On top of this, there is not always a distinct cut-off point where our heightened abilities suddenly change (although this can happen). More often our abilities gradually build at the beginning of the phase and then slowly evolve into the abilities of the next phase. All our planning can seem to be blown out of the water by a cycle which is a few days too short or a week longer than usual.

Flexibility means not panicking, it means accepting that the exact timing of our heightened abilities has changed, and based on our awareness and experience, looking at how we can use the abilities of the new Optimum Time to make progress. It means getting out the diary and planning for the next time the Optimum Time appears.

Let me give you an example:

At the moment of writing this section, I am on holiday in Portugal. Trying to get the best price on the flights meant that our holiday dates coincided with my *Creative* and *Reflective* phases. Although this is a holiday, 'awareness' meant that I knew my creative phase is my best time for writing, and 'trust' and 'action' meant that I had planned to use this Optimum Time to write.

Two days into the holiday I thought I'd better start writing, thinking that I had a whole week of Optimum Time ahead of me. Yes, you've guessed it – my hormones changed and I was in my *Reflective* phase seemingly way too early!

Looking back, I had known in the run-up to going away that I was ready to write, but with so much to organize before traveling I had ignored it, feeling confident of the diary dates and planning. My body, though, had been telling me that I was already in my Optimum Time.

So where does this leave me? Free to have a holiday without the pressure of writing? Not quite. I am still writing, but this time I am simply jotting down the ideas, insights and concepts coming out of my *Reflective* phase. I will then review all the scraps of paper, which now litter our holiday apartment, in my *Dynamic* phase, where I will group them together into a structure to form the core of the next chapter. In my next *Creative* phase I will then write the text, and perhaps I'll be a little more alert to the changes in my body this time.

In the meantime, I will do my deep reflective thinking stretched out on the beach!

Hopefully you can now see how the five keys work together. Throughout the Optimized Woman Daily Plan I will give you ideas on the type of practical action you can take in tune with your Optimum Times; however, if your Optimum Time changes unexpectedly like mine did, you can always skip forward in the plan.

The more you put your heightened abilities into action, the more conscious you will become of what you can do, and the more flexible you will become in the way you approach problems, tasks and goals. Rather than regretting the passing of a heightened skill, or wishing that you could always have this level of skill, you will instead be asking yourself how you can apply your new Optimum Time abilities to the present task. You may even achieve greater insights and accomplishments than you would have if you were simply 'consistent' all the time.

Summary

- You can start the plan immediately.
- To help get the most from the plan, it is useful to recognize the best approach, to understand more about the cycle, and to have an idea of the types of heightened abilities experienced and how they can be applied.
- **Awareness** of our physical, mental and emotional changes throughout the month helps us to discover when our heightened abilities occur, and may even lead to our discovering new talents!
- **Being self-aware** not only helps us to achieve more and do better but it also builds self-confidence and self-esteem.
- **Planning** for our phases of heightened ability enables us to match tasks to the appropriate Optimum Time, releasing our full potential, producing the best result, and getting tasks done quickly and efficiently.
- **The plan** becomes a powerful tool to achieve success and personal fulfillment, used alongside our diary.
- Taking the right **action** in the right Optimum Time enables us to experience for ourselves the power and variety of our heightened abilities. Potential talents become actual skills.
- **Experiencing** our abilities by taking action will make us more willing to leave tasks until the appropriate Optimum Time, because we will know how much easier and quicker it will be.
- **Trusting** our heightened abilities comes from enjoying the sometimes amazing results of applying them practically to the goals and tasks we have at the time, and from the confi-

dence of knowing, through 'awareness', of when they arise or change.

- Being **flexible** and able to adapt when things don't go to plan means acknowledging that our heightened abilities are cyclic phases, and deciding how the heightened skills we are experiencing can be best applied to the task at hand.
- We will always have **another opportunity** for a particular heightened ability in the following month.

"Optimized Woman allows a woman to understand why she is not consistent but rather cyclical. With this awareness, she can use her Optimum Times of energy, creativity, relationship building and alone time to benefit her health, her family and her career. I am deeply grateful to Miranda for her inspiring work." Zahra Haji, Yoga Goddess, Canada.

Chapter 3

Getting to know your phases

The body's cycle

Most of us know that our menstrual cycles revolve around two peak times; the release of the egg at ovulation, and the release of the womb lining at menstruation.

While menstruation is obvious to all, and the pre-menstrual phase very obvious to those who experience PMS, fewer women are aware of their changes in the pre-ovulation phase and at ovulation. The lack of awareness of these phases creates the false impression that menstruation is a single event repeating monthly rather than one phase in a cycle of monthly changes.

> **The body's monthly cycle**
> **Menstruation:**
> Approximately days 1-5:
> The womb sheds the old lining
> **Pre-ovulation:**
> Approximately days 6-11:
> An egg develops in the ovaries, the womb lining thickens and hormone levels rise.
> **Ovulation:**
> Around days 12-16:
> An egg matures and is released ready for fertilizing.
> **Pre-menstrual:**
> Approximately days 17-28:
> Hormone levels drop. A fertilized egg will embed itself in the womb lining.

Where we experience painful or disruptive PMS and menstrual symptoms we can gain the impression that we are 'normal' most of the time but suffer a condition which makes us 'abnormal' for a number of days a month. Seeing the menstrual cycle in this way means that we lose the concept of a 'cycle'. It becomes defined as a single abnormal event which repeats throughout our diaries.

We fail to recognize that we interpret 'normal' for women as 'abnormal'. We also miss out on recognizing that there are phases to the cycle which manifest in everyday life as different ways of thinking, different skills and abilities, and different needs. We also lose the opportunity to be aware that our cycle is a constant flow of changes and that we never stop in our process of becoming the next phase or leaving the last phase of who we are.

In general, we really don't appreciate that we are not the same person one week to the next, and tend to be unaware of many of our body's changes and their effect on our thoughts, our abilities, our feelings and our needs.

> "Really surprised, when reading back, how I change throughout the month."
> Melanie, Teacher, UK.

For example, our pain thresholds change throughout the month. Our vision and hearing can alter, our heart rate, physical stamina, co-ordination and spatial awareness, breast size and consistency, urine composition, body temperature and body weight can all vary.

These many different changes affect not just our physical energy and stamina and the way we think but also the relationship between our conscious and subconscious levels of awareness. Our behavior, skill sets, sexuality and spirituality can all change throughout the month, yet we have been taught to expect to be the same person with the same attributes all the time.

From nature's point of view, the menstrual cycle is there to restore our fertility each month. It gives us the opportunity to become pregnant. The physical, mental and emotional changes we undergo are designed to get us ready for pregnancy; but when pregnancy doesn't occur, the changes created by the menstrual cycle have a different but equally important role. Unfortunately it's this role which goes unrecognized by the current limited view of the purpose of the menstrual cycle.

If a child doesn't develop, or we already have children, or we don't want to have a family, the changes inherent within the menstrual cycle are there for us to create life in another way. They are there to help us to create relationships, community, structure, growth, goals and plans, success and achievement, harmony, art, religion, science and the future.

Our cycle is a powerful resource of skills and abilities designed for women to create culture and society, and it is our culture and society which will nurture the future generations and create the future. But the cycle is not only altruistic, it provides women with the skills and aptitudes to make a mark in the world, to achieve and create personal success and fulfillment. Nature doesn't just want us to be breeding machines; instead she supports us in our individuality and in our goals and dreams through the different abilities within the four phases of the menstrual cycle.

> **In essence, the menstrual cycle is there for us to create society and culture, and to support us in our individual goals and dreams.**

What do you mean I change each month?

I have been talking so far about the 'four phases' of the menstrual cycle but these phases do not have rigid barriers; the demarcation is simply there to help us compare and contrast each week. In the Optimized Woman Daily Plan, subdividing the cycle into defined phases makes it easier for us to compare phases and discover changes which may be difficult to identify on a daily basis.

The phases are actually experienced as a gradual change from one set of energies, abilities and perceptions to another. For example, the beginning of the *Expressive* phase (ovulation phase) will be a blend of our *Dynamic* phase (pre-ovulation phase) abilities and energies with our *Expressive* phase attributes. The *Dynamic* phase abilities will be lessening as the *Expressive* phase abilities strengthen.

This can seem very confusing at first, but there are two models we can use to make it a little easier to understand the flow of the menstrual cycle and to help us become aware of the changes in ourselves.

When we look at our cycles, we discover two phases that seem to be more action and 'doing' focused, and two phases which are experienced as more passive and more aligned with 'being'. We also notice that there are two phases which are more external world and reasoning orientated and two which are subconscious world and intuition focused.

The active-passive model of the menstrual cycle

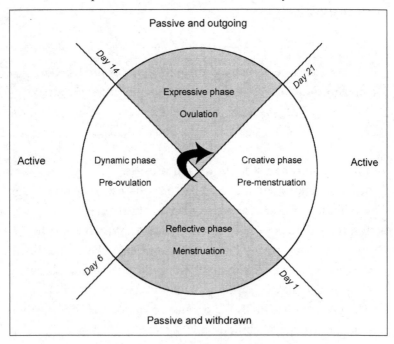

Figure 2 The active / passive cycle.

In our menstrual cycles we can experience two phases which are more action focused and ego-led – the *Dynamic* phase (pre-ovulation) and the *Creative* phase (pre-menstruation). In the *Dynamic* phase we can experience a renewed spark of physical energy after menstruation, and the drive, willpower and self-motivation to make things happen. We experience a strong need or desire to make changes and take action, but as we draw closer to the *Expressive* phase this need starts to lessen and we become more accepting of situations.

Similarly in the *Creative* phase we often experience strong bursts of physical activity and a driving need to create or 'do something'. This need for action often comes with increasing frustration as our physical stamina starts to decline the closer we get to the Reflective phase.

One way of understanding the menstrual cycle is to think of it in terms of tides. The *Expressive* phase is our high tide, the *Reflective* phase our low tide, and the *Dynamic* and *Creative* phases are the action currents of the incoming and outgoing tides.

The *Expressive* phase and the Reflective phase, like the high and low tides respectively, are more passive phases. They lack the urgent zeal to make things happen, but rather offer a gentler and more accepting, patient and nurturing approach. The *Expressive* phase brings groundedness and a welcome rest from the driving power of our will and ego. Like the high tide, the *Expressive* phase is brimming with fullness and potent energy, which allows us to support others, create relationships and connect in an empowered way with the outside world.

The *Reflective* phase is our low tide; it's a time when our physical energy and our drive and ego withdraw. It's only by the withdrawal of the water at low tide that room is made for the new waters of the future incoming tide. It's our time to rest, to let go of the cares of the world and to recharge our energies.

Let's take a walk through a cycle to see how this model is experienced in everyday life, and how we can practically use these Optimum Times.

The action-focused and passive you:

1. Reflective phase: Passive
Approximately days 1- 6 (during the menstrual 'period')

Menstruation is a time when we can experience lower physical stamina, an increased need for sleep, and the lessening of our mental ability to focus and recall. We may find that we can't face activity, or it takes added willpower and effort to take action. We can even find ourselves staring out of the window in a daze, unconnected to the world and the sense of urgency which normally fuels our day.

We can find ourselves more accepting and tolerant and more able to compromise and to let go of our desires and needs.

This passive phase is the Optimum Time to slow down, to nurture our bodies and give them the space to rest and renew. It is the time to let go of all our cares, to simply be who we are in the present moment, to be creative through day-dreaming, to go with the flow, and to reconnect with what is important to us.

2. Dynamic phase: Active
Approximately days 7-13

Once our menstruation starts to end, we emerge from our hibernation-like state. Our body no longer feels sluggish, and has much more energy and stamina. Once again we feel motivated to get active both physically and mentally.

With our sharper intellect,

> "(*Day 8. Dynamic phase*) Attention span and focus good. Multi-tasking easier. People management skills – active listening and validation come easier. Ability to think logically." Déborah, Fashion House Assistant Stylist, France.

tasks which we couldn't face during menstruation can be done quickly, and we are more able to make clinical and logical choices. We can feel a strong urge to make changes in the world to fulfill our need for action, impact, results and control, and to make things happen the way we want.

This active phase is obviously the Optimum Time to start new lifestyle regimes, to make changes in our life and work, to start new projects, and to initiate action.

3. The Expressive phase: Passive
Approximately days 14-20

As we enter the time around ovulation our levels of physical stamina, willpower and drive gradually start to change. We become less action-orientated, less assertive, and less determined to get our projects completed and our personal needs fulfilled. We can become gentler, more aware of other people's needs, and more able and willing to connect with them and to support them.

We still have a good level of physical energy, but unlike the *Dynamic* phase our emotions and emotional relationships become more important.

This phase is the Optimum Time to support projects rather than to drive them, to make new connections with people and to create outcomes as a team rather than as an individual. For some women and cultures, the energies and abilities of this phase define the meaning of being female.

4. The Creative phase: Active
Approximately days 21-28

The *Expressive* phase gradually flows into the phase which many women find the most difficult; the pre-menstrual phase.

Like the *Dynamic* phase, we are more self-orientated and we can experience a lot of active desire and drive to do things. Unlike the *Dynamic* phase, this can be a phase of

> "Last month I went through all my stuff and cleared out three bags of rubbish. It wasn't until I checked my dates that I found I was in my Creative phase!" Yassmin, Legal assistant, UK.

reducing physical energy and stamina, and of strong emotions and passions.

Our ability to create in this phase is not just limited to creating things, but also includes mental creativity. However be aware that our thinking processes can easily get out of control making us feel anxious and fearful, needy, judgmental and critical.

Surprisingly, this can be the most potent Optimum Time. It's a great time for using intolerance to fuel the clearing out of mental, emotional and physical debris. It's amazing how many women go through frantic cleaning and tidying a few days before menstruation! The mind's ability to create, extrapolate and imagine makes this a powerful time for blue-sky thinking, 'Eureka' moments and inspired ideas.

Finally, as we enter the menstrual phase, we slow down physically, mentally and emotionally, to allow ourselves to renew.

You can see from this walk through the cycle that there are times when we can experience more action-focused energies and times when our energies are more passive. It therefore makes sense to use the action phases for making things happen and the gentler, passive phases for supporting and nurturing our projects, ourselves and our relationships.

When we expect to have active phase energy and abilities during a passive phase, we can create a great deal of internal tension, frustration and stress. Similarly, being forced to be passive, patient and empathic in an action-focused phase can also create stress. In both cases we are fighting to force ourselves to be something we are not.

> **When we grant ourselves the freedom to be who we are, whatever phase we are in, we generate feelings of self-acceptance, validation and self-confidence.**

Matching our actions and expectations to the flow of action and the passive phases in our cycle can release us from the internal stress of fighting ourselves and generate feelings of self acceptance, self worth and validation.

Seeing the menstrual cycle separated into two action-focused and two passive energy phases is not the only way we can view our cycles. We can also see the cycle as a flow between our outer world, conscious awareness and our inner world, subconscious awareness.

The conscious and subconscious model of the menstrual cycle

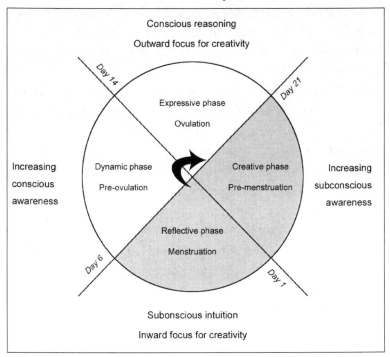

Figure 3 The conscious / subconscious cycle.

When we look at our experiences throughout the month, we notice that we can divide the cycle into two halves; one more focused on rational thought and the external world, and one where we are more focused internally on our intuitive and subconscious world.

The two externally focused phases, where our thoughts and awareness are more focused on the outside world and rational thought processes are stronger, are the *Dynamic* phase (pre-ovulation) and the *Expressive* phase (ovulation).

The two internally focused phases where our subconscious and intuitive world awareness is stronger are the *Creative* phase (pre-menstruation) and the *Reflective* phase (menstruation).

We can use the image of the moon's phases to help us understand this division. The *Dynamic* and *Expressive* phases are the increasing (waxing) and full phases of the moon, where light and the outer or visible world is dominating or dominant.

The *Expressive* phase is the peak of our shining out into the world.

The *Creative* and *Reflective* phases are the decreasing (waning) and hidden phases of the moon, where darkness and the unseen world of the subconscious and intuition are dominating or dominant.

The *Reflective* phase is our time to withdraw into the depths of our being beneath everyday thought. Like the moon, we travel between the realms of light and darkness, of rational thought and subconscious awareness.

This may sound a bit 'out there', but it's key to understanding and using the powerful Optimum Times in our cycles to create not only fulfillment, well-being and success, but also to discover and use amazing talents we never knew we had.

My awareness of my cyclic abilities came from my work. I never considered myself as a writer; I was an artist first and foremost, someone who thought in images and not words. However, I discovered that in my pre-menstrual phase I can write. When I am 'in the zone', the words flow easily and what I write is a constant surprise to me, especially when I read it back in another phase.

It is a beautiful and wondrous gift and one I never knew I had until I started not to look for consistency, but to look at my inconsistency and see what I could do with it. I hope that as you work with the Optimized Woman Daily Plan you will find your own surprise gifts!

> **When you look not for consistency but at what you can do with your inconsistency be prepared to be surprised!**

So how is this model experienced in everyday life, and how can we practically use these Optimum Times?

During the *Creative* and *Reflective* phases, where the subconscious becomes more immediate than the conscious mind, we are much more likely to experience those

> "(*Reflective phase*) A time for dreaming and planning for a future time." Natasha, Library Assistant, UK.

amazing intuitive 'Eureka' moments where ideas, creative solutions and realizations spring apparently out of nowhere.

In the *Creative* phase, with its drive and energy, we can experience the amazing ability to pull concepts out of the ether, make connections, passionately communicate our beliefs, ideas and designs, and run with an idea so far outside the box that people can't keep up. Is this an exciting time? You bet!

So often the *Creative* phase is seen as negative because of the emotional and mental disruption, but it is a powerful phase for change, growth and healing.

During this phase, as the subconscious becomes more dominant our repressed and blocked emotions and mental issues seep through into everyday awareness. Suddenly we experience emotions and thoughts that can seemingly appear out of nowhere.

However, rather than being negative, this creates a powerful Optimum Time to discover our deepest issues. It offers us the opportunity to be aware of issues our subconscious needs us to validate and process for positive growth and well-being.

Following the *Creative* phase, the *Reflective* phase can seem gentler and we can experience interacting with everyday life on a completely different level. We have a greater awareness of our inner knowing, and our intuition can be stronger than our ability to reason and to think logically.

As in the *Creative* phase, insights and ideas come out of nowhere, but we often lack the drive and energy to act on them and they tend to consist of deep insights rather than things to create in the external world. In the *Reflective* phase, the ego is quieter and we have a chance to see who we are beneath our everyday thoughts, fears, and expectations.

Both these phases are ideal for personal development, clearing the past, validating and releasing our emotions, expressing our creativity, re-framing the way we think, realizing what in our lives really fits in with our true feelings and aspirations, and for getting in touch with our intuition.

The other two phases in the cycle, the *Dynamic* phase and the *Expressive* phase are more dominated by rational thought processes and the outside world. It's not enough to have a great idea; we need to work out what to do with it and how to structure or apply it. The *Dynamic* phase allows us to do just that.

In this phase our creativity can be much more mentally-oriented, enabling us to think things through logically, apply ideas in a practical way, create working concepts, problem-solve in a methodical approach, and to see the larger picture while recognizing and creating detail.

In the *Expressive* phase, how we connect, communicate and relate to the outside world becomes important. Our sense of self and purpose so often becomes wrapped up in others in this phase, and our feelings of worth and achievement depend on our relationships with others and with the world. In the *Reflective* phase, our sense of individuality and achievement can seem quite nebulous.

The *Expressive* phase is an opportunity to build relationships which will support us and our projects, to make connections, and to communicate and present our ideas to those who can make them happen.

These two models of looking at the cycle, the Active and Passive model and the Conscious and Subconscious model, are simply concepts to try to explain our cyclic experiences and to build some sort of structure on which to view a complex pattern. You may well come up with something very different for your own cycle. What these models do is to give us a sense of the ebb

"I believe I speak for many women that night when I say that I will never experience my cycle the same way again... your presentation really pulled the pieces together for me by providing a language and a framework from which to validate my choices and experiences". Amy Sedgwick, Registered Occupational Therapist, Red Tent Sisters, Canada.

and flow of the energies experienced each month, and help us to discover who we are and what we need to do in order to create well-being and feelings of fulfillment.

Finding Fulfillment

If we view ourselves as a consistent being, we expect to experience consistent needs and what meets our needs one week should equally meet them the following week. However, when we come to terms with our cyclic nature we suddenly realize that this expectation doesn't work for us. To be happy and fulfilled in life we need to be happy and fulfilled in each phase, and just as we have different abilities and ways of perceiving in each of the phases we also have different needs to express and to meet.

Many women find accepting their cyclic nature difficult and will have one or two phases in which they wish they could stay all the time. It's not unusual for the career woman to want to stay in her *Dynamic* phase abilities, or a mother to want to stay in her *Expressive* phase for the empathic qualities that come forward. The cry of 'Wouldn't it be fantastic if I could be like this all the time, just think of what I could achieve and be like?' is heartfelt.

If we did stay in the *Dynamic* phase, we would certainly be more active and more achievement and success-orientated. And yes, we would be more able to fight in a masculine business structure because we would think and behave more like men. But we would also lose out on encountering and expressing the wide range of skills and experiences that make us feel complete.

We would lose the natural empathy and understanding of the *Expressive* phase which make us a good 'people person', a good team player or manager, and good in customer / client interaction and support.

We would also lose the inspirational leaps of the *Creative* phase which solve problems, spark the successful ad campaign, create the connection between people and their need fulfillment, or produces the workshop, product, article, approach or computer coding which changes the lives of many for the better. And finally by losing the stillness of the *Reflective* phase we would lose the ability to know what's right for us and what we should change to bring well-being and create the life we wish to live.

If we accept that we are cyclic in nature and see the positive aspects of each of the phases, and then actively live within the monthly flow of changing awareness, energies, and fluctuating abilities and skills, we naturally give equal priority to our contrasting needs:

In our relationships and in our personal achievement.

In our home life and in our career.

In our requirement for action and empowerment and in our experience of simply 'being'.

To stop and let go and to take action to start something new.

To experience our subconscious world and to focus on our external world.

To think rationally and to acknowledge our intuition.

To be analytical and to benefit from our inspiration and creativity.

Within one cycle we can actively support and interact with all aspects of our lives and of our being, without allowing anything to dominate. We live the ultimate work-life balance, fulfilling all our wants and needs as well as our dreams and responsibilities.

And the keys to this ultimate work-life balance?

1. **Don't try to be everything at once.**
2. **Don't try to be the same throughout the month.**

Making it work for you!

To bring fulfillment into our lives we need to understand and explore the cycle's phases in a little more detail. We need to look at how the different phases can affect us, and find positive and practical ways to apply our monthly changes to our lives, work, dreams and goals.

In the next four chapters we are going to investigate some of the main changes in each phase, the impact they have on us and the opportunities they present as Optimum Times. Each chapter provides a list of the possible abilities, the approaches that may work well in this phase, the things to look out for and which may not work, physical strategies, emotional strategies and finally work and goal fulfillment strategies. There are also areas for you to add your own ideas.

You may like to re-read these chapters in the appropriate phase of your cycle, as this will help you to compare the information with your own experience and also help you to identify positive and practical ways to apply your heightened skills and abilities to your life.

Every woman's experience of her cycle is unique, but there are some experiences which many women share. Some of the abilities and actions outlined in the following chapters may actually suit a different phase for you rather than the one mentioned. There are no fixed rules to working with the menstrual cycle, so work with what fits you best.

Summary:

- Physically we go through many changes during the month, many of which we are unaware of but which have an impact on how we feel, think and behave.
- Our cycle is a constant flow of changes. The distinction of four phases is simply a tool to help us become more aware of our changes by comparing different weeks in the cycle.
- It is unrealistic to expect ourselves to be the same throughout the month when we are not.
- The menstrual cycle is designed not only for the renewal of fertility and the creation of children, but also for the creation of culture, society and individual purpose and expression.
- We can use two models to help us understand the changes in the menstrual cycle. We can see the cycle as a repeating ebb and flow of action-focused energies and passive energies, and as the movement of our awareness from the conscious external world to the subconscious intuitive world and back again.
- When we accept our cyclic nature we stop having unworkable expectations and reduce the stress we place on ourselves by fighting to remain consistent.
- Within the menstrual cycle we have a powerful tool for creating happiness, well-being and fulfillment.

- Living life in tune with each part of our cycle, means that we give equal priority to all aspects of our lives and of ourselves. We naturally meet our changing needs in each phase.
- The menstrual cycle gives us the opportunity to create long-lasting work-life balance.
- The easiest way to create this balance is to live in a way that is natural to who you are in each phase.

Chapter 4

Working with the Creative phase Optimum Time

We are going to start our investigative path through our cycle's phases with the *Creative* phase (pre-menstrual phase) because this is probably the most difficult phase for many of us, especially if we experience some of the wide range of disruptive pre-menstrual symptoms. This can be the phase that has the most impact on our working lives, on our relationships, and on how we feel about what we are doing and about ourselves.

There are many different ideas about the causes of PMS, and for some women their monthly symptoms have such a disruptive affect that I certainly would not wish to trivialize their experiences. The plan in this book can work alongside any other treatment or approaches, and creating the personal Cycle Dials outlined in *Chapter 10* can help to identify when symptoms arise and what affects them.

The *Creative* phase can be the most challenging phase; some months more so than others. We can experience an overall gradual decline in stamina and mental ability and an increase in physical tension, frustration and aggression, combined with extreme sensitivity and mood swings, and overwhelming emotions and feelings from our deepest self. It can also be

"(*Day 26. Creative phase*) Need for more sleep and less time for social niceties. Dispassionately able to kick out what doesn't work and sensitive to criticism and judgement. Lack of creative feelings and feelings of success." Déborah, Fashion House Assistant Stylist, France.

challenging for people around us to protect themselves from our restlessness, anxiety-fuelled outbursts and fault-finding, and our gradual withdrawal into our internal subconscious realm.

Would I change having a *Creative* phase? No! Why? Because it offers talents and opportunities that I don't have at any other time, such as flashes of brilliant insight and awareness, and the opportunity to clear out my emotional baggage and find out what really matters to me.

Some months, however, like everyone else, I can't wait for the hormones to shift; but these are the months when I'm not listening to my body or giving time to my subconscious needs.

Creative phase overview

The *Creative* phase starts after the *Expressive* phase with a gradual decrease in levels of physical energy and stamina and in mental concentration and recall. The closer we get to the start of the *Reflective* phase the more obvious this decline becomes.

The *Expressive* phase is focused on the external world, and this is still strong at the beginning of the *Creative* phase.

As we progress through the phase our internal world becomes more impactful as our subconscious comes closer to our conscious awareness, providing inspirational bursts and uncovering any unresolved or pressing emotional issues. We can also experience a strong drive to take action, to make changes, to put things 'right' and to create.

As our physical energies

"(*Creative phase*) I am often more energetic during this phase and my physical activity increases exponentially... I also often feel inspired to sort out filing or cupboards or give the home a really good clean ... I am often too impatient to see an idea through, although have been known to jot down ideas for later use." Yassmin, Legal Assistant, UK.

reduce and our levels of mental concentration lessen, the window of opportunity to act productively on these drives decreases, often causing increased frustration, anger and irritation.

The *Creative* phase can be experienced as a roller-coaster ride of bursts of physical action, creativity and aggression alongside times of tearfulness, emotional sensitivity and neediness, negative thoughts and imaginings, and an increasing need for rest.

We can find that being able to think in a structured way becomes difficult, but we are more able to intuit things and pull ideas, understanding and connections out of nowhere.

Summarized like this, the *Creative* phase sounds pretty extreme but in fact it offers us some wonderful, positive and powerful experiences and skills. In this phase we have the opportunity to combine deep levels of awareness with action to create, heal, bring new order, and break through the thresholds of old thinking.

The Creative phase brain

One of the amazing abilities that can arise as the *Creative* phase evolves into the *Reflective* phase is the ability to meditate. As a teacher of healing and meditation it has been obvious to me that women can reach deeper levels of meditation with ease as they near the end of their *Creative* phase. In fact for some of us we can almost find ourselves in a waking meditation.

In my first book *Red Moon* I called this experience being 'between the worlds', where although we can be aware and operate in the outside world, our perception and awareness of self is turned inward.

A paper by David Noton PhD entitled *PMS, EEG and Photic Stimulation* printed in the *Journal for Neurotherapy* in 1977 states:

"An EEG study of six women with PMS demonstrated that when they were premenstrual, their EEGs showed more slow (delta) activity ..."

Delta waves are brainwaves which occur when we slip from dreaming sleep into deep sleep. Advanced meditators are able to train their brains to produce delta waves without being asleep and experience profound peace, oneness and tranquility. Unfortunately David Noton goes on to say:

> "It is concluded that PMS belongs to a group of disorders characterized by excessive slow brainwave activity."

What he has missed is something very profound and crucial. Women have a natural experience of deep meditation at this time.

It is interesting to note that if we go searching online for information on the menstrual cycle and brainwaves, rather than a plethora of medical research supporting the idea that women's thinking abilities change, what we actually find are numerous sites selling CDs of sound frequencies which will induce particular brainwave responses for deep meditation, including delta waves.

As women we have a natural ability during our monthly cycle to reach meditation depths that bring levels of restorative relaxation any male meditator would love to achieve. And it's for free! We also have easy access

> "I seem to start this phase (*Creative phase*) quite focused and then fall into an emotional, solitary state." Natasha, Assistant Librarian, UK.

to the part of our brain that stores everything we experience, that has a greater perception of the world around us, which is aware of links and synchronicities, and which connects us to feeling a unity with everything.

Within our monthly cycle we can naturally experience deep levels of meditation and restorative relaxation.

It's difficult to hear this opportunity described as a 'disorder'; however, where this paper helps is by presenting research showing that women do actually think differently with different brainwave patterns depending on where they are in their cycle.

Another intriguing impact of our changing brain state in the *Creative* phase is on our co-ordination and spatial awareness. Many women experience 'klutziness'' during the *Creative* phase, but what they can be less aware of is the peaks of almost super-woman co-ordination and dexterity.

One way of experiencing this super power is by playing sports during the more active part of our *Creative* phase – although we shouldn't rely on stamina to help us win! The only time I ever beat my husband at sport is when I am in my *Creative* phase. All I have to do is to stop thinking consciously about what to do next and the shot goes in, or I manage to reach an 'impossible' return with lightning reflexes. Unfortunately this super co-ordinated time doesn't last long. When I go to pick something up off a shelf and knock it over, I know that the winning streak is over.

The Creative phase and puppy power!

The *Creative* phase is not called 'creative' for nothing. The subconscious has a powerful ability to imagine, extrapolate, and create reality. We can ask it to show us the projected future based on a single thought or idea, or we can ask it to extrapolate and create various ways to achieve a goal or solve a problem.

Einstein was said to get dream answers to problems he was working on while sleeping. In the *Creative* phase we have the wonderful opportunity to actively access this same brain state during the day to solve all our problems. How amazing and powerful is that?

During the *Creative* phase we have the ability to readily access the information that is processed outside of our conscious awareness. This means that what we have stored in our subconscious becomes more reachable, making us much more likely to experience creative leaps and sudden shifts in perception and realization.

We can compare the subconscious to a very enthusiastic puppy that is willing to do anything to please us. If we throw a ball for a puppy it will run after it and bring it back, plus perhaps any other balls it has found. Throw it a stick and we'll have a huge pile of sticks at our feet in no time!

> **Our subconscious is like having a very bouncy puppy that is willing to do anything to please us.**

We can put this little puppy to positive everyday use. We can deliberately send it running off in a particular direction with orders on what to bring back. For example, we can plant thoughts in the subconscious about things we wish to make progress on. We can think about a project that needs inspiration or insight, or a concept or relationship we wish to understand or explore further, or we can simply want a great idea about something!

To give you an example, when I was an illustrator I was asked to illustrate a number of insects that live on brickwork for a children's natural history book. Now I don't know about you, but I don't usually take much notice of brickwork, so I said to my puppy mind 'go fetch me some brickwork'. In the run-up to painting, wherever I went I noticed bricks; their color and texture, their sizes and type of mortar, and the way plants grew on them. My puppy mind was bringing me back exactly the information I had asked for. Two days after painting the picture and sending it off to the publishers I was still noticing brickwork, because I had forgotten to tell the puppy to stop!

The search-and-retrieve ability of our puppy mind enables us to create huge leaps in awareness and understanding, as well as producing out-of-the-box solutions and inspired ideas. Our puppy mind is able to:

- rummage through all the unconscious information we hold
- find connections that we had been unable to formulate consciously
- discover the core patterns beneath details
- point out the relevant information, opportunities and coincidences which surround us all the time.

So how do we use this puppy power? There isn't a specific way to activate this ability other than to give attention to the information or solution we would like to have, or the situation and outcome we would like to create.

This doesn't mean to worry about it, but rather to take a day-dream approach with the added knowledge that we are ready to receive ideas, solutions, and synchronous opportunities and events. The answer is unlikely to come immediately, but hey the puppy takes time looking for stuff! To use a computer metaphor, think of it as hourglass time.

The answers, solutions, or a new way of viewing a project, can come to us at any time, any place and anywhere, which is why it is important to carry a notebook and pen to jot them down. Once the puppy has dropped something at our feet, we don't actually have much time to record it. The puppy can be off searching again immediately, and we can very quickly lose the inspired idea or the words and images to communicate it effectively, especially if we are near the end of the *Creative* phase.

Unfortunately most jobs don't give us much quiet alone time for creative thinking. However the *Creative* phase is one of the most powerfully creative times for women, and a totally under-used and unmanaged business resource. Until businesses allow us dedicated creative thinking time, we need to snatch moments where we can, such as a walk at lunchtime or five minutes in the restroom, to seed the subconscious and send the puppy mind out searching for us. Don't waste this invaluable phase and its inspiration!

Using the Creative phase to create our reality

Our enhanced *Creative* phase abilities can also be taken one step further and actively used to help us to create the reality we desire. When we focus on the details of what we want during this phase, we build a very powerful tool for creating it.

In *Write it Down, Make it Happen*, Henrietta Klauser suggests that by writing down our desires we activate the information-processing part of our brain to start recognizing the opportunities around us. She suggests that the simple task of using our imagination to visualize our goals and writing them down gives us the power to make it happen.

We can obviously use this technique and other manifesting methods such as those mentioned in *The Secret* by Rhonda Byrne and *The Cosmic Ordering Service* by Barbel Mohr, throughout the month; but applying some of them in the *Creative* phase can make them more impactful and powerful.

One technique that is often suggested for making changes to our lives is the use of positive affirmations. Positive affirmation is a well-known self-development technique for changing our thoughts by repeating positively worded statements. We would expect that the *Creative* phase would be the Optimum Time to send our puppy mind out to collect everything to support these positive thoughts about ourselves. Interestingly, it doesn't seem to work that way. If, in the *Creative* phase, we try sending our puppy mind after a thought such as 'I am successful - everything I do builds my success', what seems to come back is 'You have got to be joking!'

Rather than the puppy bringing us back the positive thoughts, memories and viewpoints which support the thought, instead we are given fifty reasons, memories, and resistant beliefs on why this statement could not possibly be true. In this situation the puppy mind is bringing us back all the thoughts and memories from our subconscious library which oppose the new thought form and which need accepting and releasing before we can change.

This example shows how some self-development techniques may not work in the same way for women as they do for men throughout the month. In the case of positive affirmations the result can actually generate a negative or overwhelming effect if the phase is not understood.

It is important that we view our use of self-development techniques and life style changes in relationship to the phases of our menstrual cycles. Any failures may be due to the technique or change being implemented in the *wrong phase* rather than a failure of the technique itself. It can be far more productive and effective for women to use positive affirmations in the *Dynamic* and *Expressive* phases.

> **Your phases can impact on self-development techniques. Use techniques which seem in tune with the phase rather than using a single technique throughout the month.**

The Creative phase and understanding ourselves

The way we connect with the subconscious in the *Creative* phase is not all one way, with 'us' accessing 'it'. Our subconscious also impacts on our everyday thinking. It's this aspect of the *Creative* phase that can have a huge influence on our thoughts, emotions, moods, and behavior, and on our ability to create the success and effective working practice that we want.

It's not uncommon to find circumstances which are acceptable during the rest of the month to become suddenly intolerable and the trigger for emotional outbursts during the *Creative* phase. In these situations our subconscious is giving us in a big neon sign telling us that there is something here that we need to work out in ourselves.

Notice I said 'work out in ourselves'. Anything that comes up during the *Creative* phase is about **us**, and not about the other person or the situation. This is not the time to sit down and battle out our relationship problems at work or at home, but rather it is the time to sit down, turn inwards and uncover the underlying cause of our reactions. This is the time to be really truthful with ourselves as we have the unique opportunity to delve into our deepest patterns of fear, desire and need, and to understand, accept and heal difficult aspects of ourselves. We also have the opportunity to identify what is missing in our current lives that would make us feel safe and fulfilled and to take action on this knowledge in forthcoming *Dynamic* phase.

> **The Creative phase gives us the opportunity to understand, accept and heal our deepest patterns of fear, desire and need.**

The *Creative* phase can be extremely emotional, and these emotions are often initiated by our mental programming, memories and the rejected aspects of ourselves lying deep within our subconscious. These patterns need to be acknowledged, accepted and experienced if we are to release them and create healing, well-being and personal growth.

During the *Creative* phase, our subconscious uses its close relationship to our conscious mind plus its powerful ability to extrapolate and create dramatic and emotion-filled scenarios to bring our core issues to the attention of our everyday mind.

We can use the image of a rolling snowball to show how

thoughts and emotions can develop in the *Creative* phase. Imagine that we have made a snowball on a mountain top and placed it at our feet. The snowball represents our initial thought. In a work situation it could be, 'He's overlooked me for promotion yet again!'

With this thought, we gently nudge the snowball with our foot so that it starts rolling a little. With our next thought of, 'He dislikes me! He's never said a good thing about my work', the snowball gathers more snow, more energy, and suddenly as it starts to speed down the mountainside we lose control of it.

We continue to think, 'I'm such a failure. Look at all the times I haven't got promotion and been turned down for a job. I never get anything I ask for ...' and we start a long list of memories from our working life, our home life and our childhood, all supporting this thought. Now the snowball is enormous and traveling fast, gathering snow, rocks, trees and the odd innocent skier. There is no way to stop it. The final thoughts of, 'I am totally useless. I'll never make it in life' sends the avalanche crashing down on to the village in the valley below.

All these thoughts are creative extrapolations. They are messages, not reality, but we have emotionally bought-in to the thoughts we are creating, and we act on them as if they are real. This example situation could result in feelings of anger and the intention to 'have it out' with the boss as emotions, old patterns and memories of past events overwhelm our reasoning and relationship skills.

The *Creative* phase demands to be taken seriously because it is crucial to creating well-being, happiness and fulfillment. There are two positive approaches on how to handle the emotional avalanche. We can either manage our thoughts to save the village, or we can use this experience to clear out the emotional baggage from the subconscious and see it as a positive and empowering way of personal growth and development.

Whichever of these two approaches we choose to use, we need

to keep in mind that the original trigger has come from deep within ourselves as a message to our conscious awareness that something needs to be realized, experienced and acted upon.

The 'Don't kick the snowball!' approach to emotional avalanches

The first approach, 'Don't kick the snowball!', is a situation management method. It sounds easy, but unless you are reading this section during your *Creative* phase you will not truly appreciate how hard this is to do.

It can be very difficult to step back and say to ourselves, 'That's just a thought, I'm not buying in to that', partly because we think our thoughts are always right, but particularly because they appear so quickly that we have reacted to them emotionally before we realize that the thought is just that – a thought. The thoughts which create the avalanche have no more reality than imagining a pink penguin called Percy! (Bet you now have the image in your head!).

When we enter the *Creative* phase we have to be very aware that our thoughts about work, goals, life plans, co-workers, careers, what we are capable of, what we have achieved and how successful we are, are all subject to creative extrapolation by the subconscious. For example, this is not the time to take a co-worker to task about an error, because our subconscious will use this opportunity as a way to get our attention by making it into a drama out of proportion to reality.

During the Creative phase we need to be very aware that our thoughts are the subject of creative extrapolation by the subconscious. They are a message, not reality.

The *Creative* phase is also not the time to carry out major decisions like leaving your job, or confronting a boss or a client about a grievance. However, we mustn't miss the message hidden in our initial reaction; it could be that the desire to leave our job comes from feelings of a lack of recognition or a lack of creative expression or power. We need to give ourselves the *Reflective* phase to review the situation and then, if necessary, take action in the *Dynamic* phase when we are less likely to feel everything emotionally and are more able to think logically. We may still need to leave our job, but we may also find other ways to fulfill the things we are lacking in our work.

> Our Creative phase is like a huge neon sign, written by the subconscious, to alert us of something we are missing. We can ignore it, but if we do we lose out on a huge opportunity to create happiness and fulfillment in our lives.

Crossing our thresholds:

The second approach to the snowball is to let everything happen, but not take any external action. It takes courage to allow ourselves to experience all the intense emotions bottled up behind the thoughts and memories. It can hurt, make us cry, and make us want to leave it well alone.

To experience the 'avalanche' we need to have a 'safe' place where we can spend time going through these emotions without them impacting on anyone around us (the odd skier and the village inhabitants).

To sit with our thoughts and emotions and to simply allow them to be okay can seem overwhelming; the book *The Sedona Method* by Hale Dwoskin offers excellent support for working with negative thoughts in this way.

There is also another aspect to this approach to the *Creative* phase that has huge self-development implications. In his book *Thresholds of the Mind*, Bill Harris examines the concept of the human mind having a threshold level beyond which it becomes overwhelmed. He suggests that when situations get stressful we find coping methods to relieve the tension so that we don't go over this threshold. We can find ourselves eating more comfort foods, drinking more alcohol, or engaging in other stress releasing activities.

Bill Harris states however that if we allow ourselves to become overwhelmed by the experiences our mind is no longer able to hold the same patterns, and breaks down to create new patterns and behaviors. The more we go through our thresholds, the more our mind is able to adapt so that each threshold becomes higher and higher until it becomes very difficult to overwhelm us.

In the *Creative* phase our cycle can naturally create opportunities for us to cross our thresholds and take the next leap forward in self-growth. To work this way with our *Creative* phase takes courage and willpower, and also requires support. It's not something attempted lightly, and I recommend that any readers attending counseling check first with their counselor before using this approach.

> "I now welcome and embrace the more heavy energies of pre-menstruation and menstruation instead of fighting against them and feeling badly that I am not full of energy and enthusiasm throughout the month. I love and accept my cyclical nature – Thank you Miranda for this understanding." Zahra Haji, Yoga Goddess, Canada.

The concept is not to disrupt our lives in this phase but rather to help us use the opportunities our cycle offers for our benefit and advantage.

The *Creative* phase is clearly the Optimum Time for working with our subconscious for personal growth. We are given the opportunity to consciously interact with and clear out any emotional or mental habits, patterns, memories, and attitudes that we don't wish to take with us into the next phase.

This is quite a powerful statement. This phase empowers us to change the 'self' we take into the next month. Why carry all the emotional baggage we have been picking up this month into the next month? In the next month we could experience the real person hidden under all those emotional suitcases!

> **The Creative phase gives us the opportunity to drop our emotional and mental baggage so we don't have to take it into the next month.**

The Creative phase Optimum Time

The *Creative* phase offers us enhanced abilities and skills which we can use to improve our lives and our career and work, and to help us achieve our goals. To make sure that we use the phase productively we need to create strategies to ensure that we don't miss out on our enhanced abilities and develop coping tactics for tasks which we can't do quite so well.

The next section offers some suggestions and guidance on actions which can support you through the *Creative* phase and help you to use this time to work to your strengths. Reading this section in the *Creative* phase may well spark many more ideas, and there is space at the end of the chapter to record them.

Creative phase abilities:
- Excitement-led creativity – putting energy into things which inspire and ignite the fire within!
- Creative writing and communicating from the passion of the heart.
- Enthusiasm-led design, visual creation and imagination.

- Creating music from a zest for life.
- Manifesting our goals and wildest desires.
- Recognizing the hidden opportunities and synchronicities around us.
- Creating new ideas out of little information, and brainstorming.
- Blue-sky thinking and running with creative concepts.
- Making leaps in understanding.
- Magically pulling ideas out of nowhere.
- Intuitively understanding complex theories.
- Coalescing a structure out of amorphous information.
- Intuiting the core pattern behind details.
- Identifying and dropping anything unworkable or outmoded.
- Identifying problems and inefficiencies.
- Tidying to make space and order.
- Clearing out emotional baggage, old attitudes, mental behaviors and patterns to create new order.
- Knowing what looks and feels 'right' to create the effect you want.

What doesn't work so well in the Creative phase:

- Understanding something logical or thinking rationally.
- Working out problems with other people.
- Empathy.
- Teamwork.
- Starting new projects, lifestyles or regimes.
- Structured learning, thinking or planning.
- Positive affirmations about yourself and your life.
- Trying to fix yourself or your relationships.

Things to watch out for in the Creative phase:

- Mood swings.
- Experiences of irritability and intolerance, then tearfulness

and extreme empathy and emotional sensitivity.
- Being overly sensitive to criticism.
- Difficulty in being objective about information, tasks, situations and people.
- The need to be right and to be validated as right.
- A tendency to extrapolate and 'create' scenarios beyond reason.
- 'Drama Queen' actions.
- Judgmental and critical attitude reflecting excessive internal self-judgment.
- Aggression and anxiety powered by deep-rooted fears.
- Poor memory recall.
- Periods of active, fiery mental, emotional and physical energy and periods of low, sluggish energy.
- Low blood-sugar moments.
- A greater likelihood of changing your appearance in this phase than in any other.
- Don't expect others to know how to handle you. If you know, give them some guidelines and keep them updated.
- Lack of patience and tolerance; expecting things done immediately.
- Expecting others to know what you need.

Creative phase strategies:
Physical
- Take 'power naps' or meditation breaks during the day, especially towards the end of the phase.
- Get more sleep towards the end of the phase and change your lifestyle to suit this. You can catch up socially in the *Dynamic* and *Expressive* phases.
- Use extra caffeine only when really necessary. This is your body's natural time to slow down, so honor it.
- Snack on healthy foods to keep sugar levels stable.
- Use exercise to release frustration and physical stress.

- Let go of gym targets.
- When you have the physical energy, enjoy the heightened, intuitive coordination to win at sports.

Emotional

- Take time to ask your subconscious what it needs you to feel, acknowledge, release or do.
- Create 'down' time to experience and clear your old emotional patterns and thoughts.
- Write down your emotions, your dreams and desires.
- Acknowledge and feel any emotions as they appear. Try not to suppress them or act on them. Don't build the emotion with additional thoughts, memories or images; stay with the original thought (don't kick the snowball!).
- Commit to using this as a phase of positive emotional growth and change.
- To feel better, put your creative energies into action. It doesn't matter what you do, just do something fun!
- Accept your emotions and thoughts as messages from your subconscious and not as reality.
- Don't believe your negative thoughts, especially those about yourself.
- Avoid major decisions; don't take action until the Dynamic phase.
- Avoid arguments and confrontation; leave them until the Dynamic or Expressive phases.
- Don't worry when you are unable to do things in your normal way. This is not a permanent state, it will pass.
- Stay in the 'Now' – ignore the past and the future.
- Concentrate on one thing at a time to avoid panic or frustration.
- Give up, give in, and surrender.
- Look after your own needs so you don't get angry when others don't meet them for you.
- Avoid people who are negative, depressive or needy.

Work

- Enjoy creative blue-sky-thinking time to focus on positive solutions and 'Eureka' ideas.
- Have fun throwing the ball for the 'puppy mind' while taking a walk or spending an extra five minutes in bed.
- Keep a note pad to jot down puppy mind inspirations – and everything else if your memory gets poor.
- Use your super-judgmental powers for good and focus on projects which really need critical analysis, ie. not by criticizing yourself or your co-workers!
- Keep flexible. Do things when you have the energy, don't leave it until later as you may not have the physical or mental energy at that time.
- Take a break to listen to your inner needs. What is it that your work is not meeting?
- Critically analyze your 'to do' list and cross out anything not worth doing, or that you'll never get round to.
- Focus restless energies productively into spring clearing your work area. What around you needs throwing out?
- Note what is inefficient or ineffective and create new structures and organization. Remember this is also an external sign of a need for some inner clearing.
- Believe only in the thoughts which fire enthusiasm and energy.
- Use your thought processes. Focus on ways to do things better, more economically, or more efficiently.
- Just because you have to do a task that is not suited to this Optimum Time doesn't mean you can't do it. You simply may not reach your own high levels of expectation.
- Don't feel guilty that you're not working as hard as everyone else. You are working in a different capacity, and can always catch up in the *Dynamic* phase.
- Call for help and support from other people when working on tasks which are not suited to this Optimum Time,

especially if you're unable to be objective about your work.

- Shift your workload to tasks that suit your abilities at this time. Try to catch up on other tasks in the Dynamic phase.
- Use different methods and approaches to learning and understanding concepts, eg. learn by watching and observing.
- Doing things which meet your current needs and abilities will create less stress and frustration and will enhance your self-confidence and self-worth.
- Try to concentrate on each task in hand, multi-tasking skills may not be good.
- Postpone or leave negotiations to others. You will not be at your most diplomatic.
- Be careful in working relationships as you may be very direct and lacking in patience and empathy.
- Don't follow up a grudge or a grievance; it may get blown out of all proportion.
- Leave socializing and networking until the *Dynamic* and *Expressive* phases.
- Use time management techniques to prioritize tasks, to avoid deadline stress and to use any bursts of energy to their maximum effect.
- Make relationships easier and more productive, by giving people some guidelines on how to interact with you. This gives them a better chance of getting things right, plus you won't get labeled 'moody'!

Goal fulfillment:

- Use this phase to find out what you feel about your goals and what patterns are resisting them.
- Clear out and drop actions and projects which haven't worked, haven't had the required impact or haven't produced the results you want.
- Make small changes; don't change your main goal.

- Don't compare yourself with other people's progress and successes.
- Don't make future plans based on your current feelings, but look at why you may feel the way you do.
- Seed your subconscious for ideas on what to do next and for solutions to problems and challenges. Use it or lose it!
- Validate who you are and what you are doing with your life.
- This is the major time for diets to break! You may find that your body naturally wants less food later in the *Reflective* phase, and you will have the motivation in the *Dynamic* phase to continue your diet.

The challenge:

- To surrender on all levels.
- To let go of the fears which generate the need for control.
- To accept and not 'fix' anything – especially yourself or your partner.
- To be comfortable with vulnerability.
- To love yourself as you are.

Your ideas for Creative phase activities:

Chapter 5

Working with the Reflective phase Optimum Time

For some women the physical transition from the *Creative* phase to *Reflective* phase is an easy one. For others, including myself, we can find ourselves at 4 o'clock in the morning curled up in the bathroom waiting for painkillers to dull the spasming cramps.

The physical side of starting menstruation can be difficult, but with the change in hormones comes an exciting new perspective and a fresh way of thinking about the world and ourselves. It can be a wonderful, welcome relief that the frenetic energy of the *Creative* phase has evolved into a period of deep letting go, of restfulness and peace, and of connectedness and well-being.

The *Reflective* phase is probably the most profound catalytic tool we have for changing actions and goals and our relationship to ourselves, and also for deepening our level of connection, experience and understanding of the universe and our place in it.

To actively use this tool we need to slow down. We need

> "During my menstrual flow I feel drawn deeply within. It's a time for me to gather insights and ideas, which I implement for the rest of the month."
> DeAnna, Speaker, Educator and Trainer, USA.

to accept that we can't match the pace of the world for a few days and make room for the *Reflective* phase abilities.

For many women, physical symptoms and work pressures can make this a problematic time of the month, but this time contains unique Optimum Time abilities and skills that we can pro-actively use to create well-being, acceptance and change.

Reflective phase overview

The *Reflective* phase starts around the time of menstruation. It can last a full week or only a couple of days, depending on the individual. Where the *Creative* phase is a time of slowing down, the *Reflective* phase is one of having stopped. It's a time when our bodies require rest to restore and renew the energies to be released again with the birth of a new cycle in the coming *Dynamic* phase.

We find ourselves naturally withdrawing from the social world, needing the reassurance of a safe place to curl up, and leaving responsibilities, demands, and tasks until later. We not only slow down physically, we also slow down mentally and emotionally. Our awareness turns inward and our intuitive thoughts and feelings are heightened as our connection with our subconscious is at its strongest.

In the *Reflective* phase we stand in our internal world, directly opposite the outer world awareness of the *Expressive* phase (see Figure 3 in *Chapter 3*). We are at the lowest ebb of the tide, that still point of rest before the water starts to move again gaining momentum with the incoming tide.

In this beautiful still point of rest the *Reflective* phase offers us the opportunity to let go of worries and concerns, simply because we don't have the energy to bother with them. The experience of deep stillness is seductive and necessary, and when we try to fight it off with willpower and caffeine we react to everyday demands with irritability, frustration and anger. To gain the active energy of the *Dynamic* phase we need our rest and stillness to restore and regroup.

The *Reflective* phase can feel like a 'living' meditation. When we think of the word 'meditation' we tend to think of someone staring at a candle for hours, a woman balancing in some extreme yoga position, or the deeply enigmatic eyes of a Buddha statue. For most of us, these images seem so far away from our everyday inner turmoil that we think we could never reach that level. However, there is an amazing gift for women in the *Reflective* phase. Meditation isn't something that we need to do, it is something we are!

> **In the Reflective phase meditation isn't something that we do, it is something we are!**

In the *Reflective* phase we naturally reach deep levels of physical and mental relaxation. Rather than fight this experience, we can instead simply enjoy our natural ability to let go and leave aside our ego self and gain the benefits of stress relief and well-being that meditation can bring.

The *Reflective* phase is also the Optimum Time to review our lives and goals to see whether they are still in keeping with who we are and what we want to achieve. Reviewing in this phase is not an analytical process but one with an emphasis on our feelings and intuitions. We can try ideas, projects, plans and dreams on for size to help our subconscious to accept and adapt to any changes we wish to make.

We're also better able to identify and acknowledge our innermost needs without self- judgment or criticism.

The *Reflective* phase is the phase to connect with our authentic self, the aspect of ourselves which lies beneath our emotional and mental patterns, and to use its guidance to shape our lives in the month ahead.

The impact of the Reflective phase

With the demands we place on ourselves, and with the expectations of the working environment, we very rarely have the luxury to let go and be true to ourselves in this phase. So often it is the extra Espresso and sheer mental determination that keeps us going. But imagine what it would be like to go without sleep and to keep going on caffeine for a few days. We would hardly be functioning at our full potential.

Every month by 'keeping going' we deny the rest our cycle, mind and body require to renew. We lose out not only on our natural ability to restore ourselves but also on our ability to access understanding, inspiration and guidance through our intuition.

> "(*Reflective phase*) I find myself 'zoning out' on these days. I am generally quite happy with life and have a philosophical outlook. I also feel particularly feminine whilst menstruating and am more inclined to be seen in a skirt rather than trousers, and may even start taking more care of my plants or cooking more." Yassmin, Legal Assistant, UK.

Our natural need to withdraw, nurture and restore ourselves impacts on all aspects of our lives whether we're conscious of it or not. In the work place, when we simply can't keep going, we have to take time off. Unfortunately this has a negative impact on the perception of women's worth as employees, women's commitment to their jobs, their ability to be reliable, and their earnings.

A report entitled *Biological Gender Differences, Absenteeism and the Earning Gap* by Andrea Ichino and Enrico Moretti (*NBER Working Paper No. 12369, July 2006*) states:

> "… *evidence that the menstrual cycle raises female absenteeism. Absences with a 28-day cycle explain a significant fraction of the male-female absenteeism gap.*
>
> *…Finally, we calculate the earnings cost for women associated with menstruation. We find that higher absenteeism induced by the 28-day cycle explains 11.8 percent of the earnings gender differential."*

This report highlights the business world's focus on **atten-dance** rather than **productivity** to demonstrate worth, and therefore remuneration.

In this light, the *Reflective* phase can be seen as having a damaging role in a woman's working life. But what would happen if the business world focused more on productivity and allowed women three days paid leave each month, around the start of menstruation, and required longer hours afterwards? The obvious argument against this idea is that it couldn't work; that productivity would suffer and it would be unfair on the male workers. However, refreshed and re-energized women could increase productivity well beyond business expectations and become a resource of inspiration, creativity and insight at a time when businesses need to be creative and flexible to stay ahead of the game.

This idea does not imply that women are not equal to men, just that we are different, and that the male working environment may be restrictive to the full potential of our talents and abilities. Many companies offer employees 'smoking breaks' on the under-standing that they catch up on their work later in the day. There is no reason why women could not be given monthly 'health breaks' on the same basis.

> **You would think that the business world would be keen to use the full creative and inspired potential that women offer!**

Reflective phase hibernation

The *Reflective* phase can feel like a time of hibernation and withdrawal. Everything can seem to take more effort, from thinking and interacting with people to simply walking or moving. Our motivation, enthusiasm and 'get-up-and-go' naturally take a well-earned break, but this doesn't mean that we're not moving forward towards achieving our goals and dreams, but for a short while we are going with the flow instead of paddling hard.

Mentally forcing ourselves to be more active in this phase often generates anger, frustration and stress, and so it's important that we find ways of dealing with demands in a way which supports this phase.

Physical and mental tiredness can cause significant problems, and it's for this reason that planning is one of the keys to using our cycles for creating success. If we start to plan tasks in our *Dynamic* phase to fit in with our Optimum Time abilities in the month ahead, we are more likely to be able to factor in the *Reflective* phase hibernation and take things at a slower pace.

One of the most impactful aspects of the *Reflective* phase is the tendency to want to be alone and to emotionally withdraw from social interaction. We can feel indifferent to people's needs and concerns, and disinterested in their ideas, projects, or work in general. Giving ourselves physical 'space' away from other workers can be supportive by reducing the number of demands on our energies and attention.

The problem with social withdrawal however is that co-workers and clients can interpret this behavior negatively as rejection, disapproval, a lack of positive validation or a lack of commitment. Rather than give people this impression we need to schedule our unavailability and to reassure that the time and effort required in the project, task or relationship will occur in a few days' time. People are very good at picking up on disingenuous behavior, so we need to postpone people-orientated tasks such as making employee appraisals, sales approaches and interviews or making new contacts and reschedule these activities for the *Expressive* phase.

As well as removing ourselves from people in order to stop

giving the wrong impression, we may also need to remove ourselves for our own protection. In the *Reflective* phase we can be so lacking in motivation and enthusiasm that we become disconnected from our own wants and needs and are unlikely to stand up for our ideas and opinions. Nothing seems important, even our own goals and ambitions. Unfortunately this can mean that we end up involved in projects or work decisions that don't suit us, because we've not made our points heard.

If we can postpone meetings until the *Dynamic* phase then not only will we care about the outcome but we will also have the self-confidence to stand up for our views, the mental ability to convince others, and the energy to create action.

The Reflective phase 'whatever' approach to self-awareness

The *Reflective* phase 'whatever' attitude makes it an Optimum Time to prioritize our lives, as nothing really has much priority. If something is really important it will be worth the effort to overcome our natural inertia, so we realize very quickly what is a 'must' action and what is a 'should'.

The *Reflective* phase naturally makes us ask the questions: 'Can I be bothered to go to work?' 'Can I be bothered to get that report completed?' 'Can I be bothered to take the children to their events?' 'Can I be bothered to clean the house?' 'Can I be bothered about anything?' 'Can I even be bothered to have goals about life and success?'

Everything can seem like too much effort when we have little energy. Rather than being a negative attitude, this can actually become a resourceful tool for self-development and goal achievement. We can look at aspects of our lives and ourselves and see if we can really be bothered to continue the current patterns of behavior and thoughts.

We have a natural opportunity to ask ourselves how important it is that we should do things; and not just the little everyday things, but the big stuff as well!

The *Reflective* phase naturally forces us to let go and stop. In the other phases we are driven by our expectations and desires, our ego and goals, and the need for movement and success to show us our worth. Suddenly this phase forces us to release the drive, but more importantly it forces us to drop our fear and anxieties. When we give up, we give up caring about the outcome, we give up buying into our expectations, needs and fears, and what other people think, and instead we simply accept the here and now.

An example is the effect exhaustion has on us. I had flown out to Jordan then taken a long coach journey through the desert to a hotel. By the time I reached the hotel at 2am I was totally exhausted. The hotel was undergoing renovations so inside was a building site, but all I could think of was a bed to sleep in. I didn't care about the mess or where my luggage was. All I wanted was something soft to lie on and a door that locked; anything else didn't matter. Exhaustion had released all the usual wants, needs, expectations and motivation down to the bare essentials of the moment.

The *Reflective* phase can be similar to this experience. If we don't have the energy to cope with the future, it disappears for us and we no longer buy-in to the expectations of what will or won't happen. Our long list of what we want or need to be happy also disappears.

This begs the question: **if we can stop caring about something through menstruation, is it still important enough for us to pick it up again in the *Dynamic* phase, or can we let it go from our life?** Some things we'll pick up again because they are habitual, but when we use this phase to consciously decide what we will drop and what we will run with, we not only add the power of deep commitment to our motivation in the month ahead but we also change who we are. We enter the new month as a new woman!

It can actually be quite difficult to explain how important and powerful the *Reflective* phase is for us when it's so alien to the modern world approach and expectations. Actively using the *Reflective* phase as a self-review tool can have a major positive impact on our well-being, happiness, confidence and attitude throughout the month ahead.

The Reflective phase ultimate self-fix

The *Reflective* phase is the Optimum Time for self-acceptance, as the natural 'whatever' attitude is also applied to us. With little mental, physical or emotional energy to 'fix' ourselves we end up accepting who we are the way we are, warts and all!

> **The ultimate self-fix of the Reflective phase is: there is nothing to fix!**

Our self-acceptance is only the shortest distance from turning into self-love, but this only happens if we mentally give in to the phase and don't try to overrule it through willpower and stimulants.

When we do let go, accept ourselves and give in to our body's need for rest, we can experience deep feelings of inter-connection with the universe, including inner peace and love. The more we allow ourselves to experience this inner connection each month the more accessible it will be to us throughout the month, allowing us to have distance from our emotions and thoughts and events.

The *Reflective* phase offers us a uniquely female path to living life from an overview perspective. It's this higher awareness of life that releases the everyday stresses, strains and tensions and opens us up to be more flexible, adaptable and loving.

If we have been under a lot of stress, or the *Creative* phase has been particularly disruptive, it can take a few days into the *Reflective* phase before we stop fighting, give in and surrender to bigger picture awareness and the 'whatever' attitude.

If we don't allow ourselves 'down time' during the *Reflective* phase, we can either take longer to develop the *Dynamic* phase energies and abilities, have less energy throughout the month, or experience physical symptoms which force us to stop. This 'down time' however is not just a case of getting more sleep or watching television. It needs to consist of active reflection.

Take time out or your body will do it for you!

Reviewing in the Reflective phase

The *Reflective* phase is the Optimum Time to turn inwards and reflect. It is the Optimum Time to ponder the previous month's events, feelings, and thoughts, to review our current projects and goals, and to commit to change.

The *Reflection* phase is very much focused on inner knowing and feeling; feeling the need for change, feeling the right type of change, and feeling commitment to that change.

Planning the details, the solutions, how and when it is going to be implemented however is best left for the optimum energies of the *Dynamic* phase. Within the phase, the Optimum Time for reflection will develop in its own timeframe. Sometimes the 'whatever' attitude of the phase will last the week, and sometimes only for a couple of days. As we gradually come out of the almost meditative experience of the *Reflective* phase we can turn our attention to reviewing, feeling, and imagining.

This is the time to ask ourselves:

'What do I feel I need to do differently?'

'What do I feel needs to change, and how?'

'What would the outcome be like? How would I feel?'

'Do I feel committed to this change? If not, is it the right change, and what could I change to make it feel right?'

This is the phase to take time to day-dream, to imagine what different scenarios would be like and how we would feel in them. We can imagine our long term goals fulfilled, short term changes, solutions to work problems and new ideas for projects. The more vividly we day-dream, the more we enhance our feelings, the more real our imaginings become to our subconscious, and the more we change at a deeper level to make it come true. In other words, the more committed we become.

As in the *Creative* phase, our subconscious will also respond to us with inspired ideas and leaps of insight. The beauty of this Optimum Time is that we can make really deep and long-lasting positive changes not only for our work and working life but also within our personality and how we interact with the world.

By using this time to reflect, we can enter the *Dynamic* phase running. We already know what needs changing in the project to make it work better (*Creative phase*), we have worked through the scenarios and are emotionally committed to it (*Reflective phase*), and we are energized to implement that change (*Dynamic phase*).

This sudden surge of enthusiasm can be a bit of a shock for co-workers who have got used to us hibernating for a few days, so it can be useful to give them a little advanced warning that in a week's time we are going to have a project shake-up!

The *Reflective* phase also offers us the opportunity to replace some of our deeper programming. In the *Creative* phase we experienced our emotions and let them go. In the *Reflective* phase we have the opportunity to process the message behind these emotions and to develop new thought patterns and beliefs. The *Creative* phase is like the Fall when we drop our emotional leaves, and the *Reflective* phase is like the winter where we decide which new leaves we will grow and where we will grow them when the spring energies return.

We are able to leave behind the effects of events in the last month and enter the *Dynamic* phase once again fresh and new. We don't have to carry the past with us; we can choose during this phase what to take and what to leave. For example, if a co-worker gave us a really hard time last month, why carry the anger into the next month to create a dysfunctional working relationship? We can leave the anger and underlying pattern behind when we touch base with our self in the *Reflective* phase, and experience self-acceptance and our place in the Universe. This means that when we once again have to work with this person we do so from a perspective of self-power, without the need for revenge or validation.

When we don't give time to acknowledging the messages of the subconscious in the *Creative* phase, the accompanying stress and tension can spill over into the *Reflective* phase, forcing us to deal with these issues before we enter the *Dynamic* phase.

It can be hard when the mind is opposing the innermost self's wants and needs to finally let go and give in to the *Reflective* phase. Sometimes the battle is so long-standing and repeated every month that we can find it difficult to give up the habit of tension, stress and fighting. It is then that we need to withdraw from the world, perhaps to lie in bed in the dark and have the courage to say 'okay, what's going on?'.

The *Reflective* phase not only offers us the opportunity to re-create who we are every month but also the ability to know what to create. When we give ourselves the space and time to withdraw and turn inwards in the *Reflective* phase, and to use our feelings as messengers from our innermost self, the *Reflective* phase becomes a beautiful, transformative and supporting time of the month.

Reflective phase opportunities

If the Reflective phase is a time of natural hibernation and inner withdrawal, what Optimum Time abilities and skills can it offer us in everyday life? Acknowledging that this can be a difficult time for women at work, what should we look out for, and what strategies can we use to make this time productive in our careers and in our goal fulfillment?

Abilities:

- The ability to forgive and forget, and to leave the past behind.
- Deep inner processing and reflection.
- Physical restoration and renewal of energies.
- Making changes, and committing to them 100%.
- Intuitively feeling the right direction or action, and the bigger picture.
- Intuitively understanding what projects, tasks, or people need.
- Natural meditative state.
- Access to subconscious ideas and information.
- Deep connection to the Universe beyond everyday concerns.
- The ability to review activities, goals and life through feelings and intuition rather than thoughts.
- Positive imagining of different futures, solutions and goals to feel if something is right, and to generate commitment.
- Enjoying deep inner feelings of peace.
- Resting the ego.
- Accepting everything as it is.
- Not being bothered by anything but the base levels of need.
- Ability to 'go with the flow'.
- Existing in the 'here and now' and not in our heads.
- Loving the simple pleasures of being.

- The ability to be happy with what you have, with no motivation to change or have more.
- The ability to be gentle with yourself and to love and accept yourself.
- Creating concepts and solutions out of the blue.
- Creative imagination.

What doesn't work so well:
- Expectations of being focused and dynamic.
- Working and networking with people; social interaction.
- Long working hours or starting new projects.
- Detailed and structure-led tasks.
- Physical activity e.g. rushing around, traveling etc.
- Learning, logical thinking or planning.
- Trying to be motivated by enthusiasm.
- Lack of sleep.
- Exercise and sporting activities.

Things to watch out for:
- Feelings of disconnection, lack of interest, and being unsociable and withdrawn.
- 'Whatever!' attitude; being too tired to make a stand.
- Lack of motivation and enthusiasm.
- The effect of withdrawal and emotional isolation on others.
- Need for nurturing.
- Don't make plans for any changes, leave the details until the Dynamic phase.
- A commitment made in your heart will change your life.
- Make time for extra sleep and relaxation.
- Over-riding or hating this natural withdrawal will create stress.
- A natural reduction in the amount we eat.
- Creating unrealistic goals and expectations for the phase.
- Not planning for this phase in the previous Dynamic phase.

- Feeling victimized or overwhelmed by others' demands and expectations.
- Impulse to drop everything, even the important stuff.
- Expecting other people to know what is going on inside you.

Strategies:

Physical

- Give the gym a break for a couple of days.
- Take naps during the day.
- Alter your routine to include more quiet time or sleep time.
- If you can organize a day in bed, do it!
- Meditate or simply rest quietly, preferably in natural surroundings.
- Use extra caffeine only when really necessary.
- Slow down. Walk slower, do less.
- Give your body simpler, healthier, unprocessed foods.

Emotional

- Withdrawal protects you from other people's emotional demands.
- Avoid major decisions. Being too tired to care may allow people to take advantage of you.
- Remember that lack of motivation and enthusiasm will pass with the start of the *Dynamic* phase.
- Reflect on the things that upset you in the *Creative* phase. Ask your subconscious for the core message and the solution.
- Don't feel guilty that you are not working as hard as everyone else; you can always catch up in the *Dynamic phase*.
- If you feel 'blissed out' enjoy it. People spend a lot of money to feel this way!
- Touch base with nature. There is a naturally supportive affinity with nature during this phase.

- Imagine different scenarios linked to difficult decisions or situations to help your subconscious to adapt, feel safe and prepared and to generate positive empowerment feelings for the month ahead.
- Trust your inner knowing and decisions to change in this phase. They will come from the deepest part of you, which will help you to commit.

Work

- Take time to review your feelings about tasks and projects.
- Day-dream about projects, tasks and problems. Don't try to force answers, simply notice your feelings.
- Trust your intuition.
- Try ideas, projects, changes, plans, goals and dreams on for size. This helps your subconscious to accept and adapt to any changes you wish to make.
- Do things outside of work which nurture and support you; say, an early evening bath with aromatherapy oils, candles, music, and chocolate!
- Still seed your subconscious for creative ideas and solutions but be aware that the response time will be slower than in the Creative phase.
- If possible avoid social and networking events. People will pick up that you are not feeling naturally extroverted.
- Give yourself permission to slow right down. Do what is necessary but no more. You can catch up later in the month.
- Be aware of when you have energy to work, and use this for tasks that need mental abilities.
- Inform co-workers that you will be less available to them for a few days.
- Reassure co-workers and clients that your lack of attention and enthusiasm over the next few days does not mean that they're not important.
- Avoid client and business meetings; you are unlikely to actively take part and may not be bothered about project

needs and wants.

- Delegate wherever possible, but only to people you fully trust; you will not have the energy or willpower to check any work.
- Keep everything simple. Do not take on too many tasks at once.
- Understand that forcing yourself to do things in this phase creates stress.
- Where possible, leave learning new skills and information to the Dynamic phase.
- For projects requiring enthusiasm and motivation from you, try to postpone involvement until the Dynamic phase.
- Remember that anything you do in this phase that is not in tune with the phase is likely to cause frustration and stress. It will also not be your best work; but then maybe you are not bothered by that!
- Don't even think about multi-tasking unless it is backed up by time management and prioritizing, and even then it may not work.
- Help people out by giving them some guidelines on how to approach you or leave you alone. Don't expect them to read your mind.

Goal fulfillment:

- Enjoy a break and simply be. Don't have any actions or tasks planned for this phase, especially at the beginning.
- Ask yourself what you have lost in the past month (or in previous months) and need to restore in order to feel fulfillment.
- Use any disruptive feelings experienced in the previous *Creative* phase as supportive guidance on active changes for the coming month.
- Decide what you are going to commit to. Be aware that a decision at this time can have some dramatic effects.

- This is the time to change your main goal if it feels wrong. Find a wording or an image or a desire that does feel completely right.
- Exercise regimes can often fall apart in this phase. This is natural, as your body wants a break to restore its energies. Don't feel guilty, simply work with your body and start afresh in the *Dynamic* phase.
- Day-dream about how you would feel if your main goal was fulfilled.
- Test out your ideas, projects and goals in your imagination. Imagine a conversation with your subconscious about them.
- In particular, test out proposed changes in your imagination to allow your subconscious to become comfortable with the idea.
- As in the *Creative* phase, you can still seed your subconscious for inspiration, but the response will be slower.
- Notice any tension or reluctance which suggests resistance, and imagine the reasons and the answer.
- In the latter part of the phase think about your goals and actions for the month ahead

The challenges:
- Accepting the phase.
- Physically stopping.
- Enjoying the phase.
- Planning to allow for 'down time'.

Your ideas for Reflective phase activities

Chapter 6

Working with the Dynamic phase Optimum Time

The *Dynamic* phase is the phase when we can get the most done – hence the name 'dynamic'! It can feel the most empowering, most productive and most rewarding phase out of the whole cycle, especially as its enhanced abilities and skills fit in with modern expectations of work and productivity. And these feelings of new energy and heightened abilities and skills are the direct outcome of the hibernation time of the *Reflective* phase. It is by allowing our bodies, minds and emotions to rest and restore themselves that we create this wonderful Optimum Time of energy and action.

The *Dynamic* phase is such a great Optimum Time for achievement, success and moving forwards that many women regret that the phase doesn't last. It is the most mentally productive phase of the whole cycle as well as the phase that can have the greatest impact on our future successes and goal achievements.

> **The Dynamic phase is the most mentally productive phase of the menstrual cycle.**

The joy of the *Dynamic* phase is the feeling it brings of self-confidence, self-belief, independence and the increased physical energy and mental clarity which empowers us to take action. This is the time to take steps and start those groundbreaking, life-changing exploits.

Dynamic phase overview

The *Dynamic* phase is the start of a new cycle and a new planning month. We emerge from the hibernation of the *Reflective* phase physically, mentally and emotionally revitalized and ready to step out into the world and make things happen. This is a really exciting phase. Our energies, enthusiasm and self-confidence are all naturally high and we are ready to start new projects, catch up on tasks left over from the previous month, and reinvent ourselves for the month ahead.

In this phase our memory is sharper, our thinking is clearer and more logical, we have greater powers of concentration and we have the ability to grasp the bigger picture as well as giving attention to fine details. We can feel a huge impetus to get things done and to take action to make changes and achieve new goals.

Physically we experience more energy, need less sleep and can stay mentally active for longer during the day, so we can work or party late into the evenings. The increased self-confidence makes us more sociable and more direct, and with these abilities plus a natural strong self-

"Over the years I came to realize that my natural gregariousness and exuberance were heightened during my pre-ovulation phase. This enhanced my work as a presenter and trainer during my 40s. I could count on being "in the zone" if I was presenting during this time, full of energy and creative ideas, and very responsive to my audience. My presentations during the other phases of my cycle weren't necessarily any less effective but required more focus and consciousness to pull off... for entertainment and energy, nothing could match my "performance" level when I was pre-ovulatory."
Laura, Executive Director, Sexual Health Access Alberta, Canada.

belief, enthusiasm and self-motivation there is nothing we feel we can't do or achieve in this phase.

We have already seen that the cycle can be viewed as a pattern of strengthening and weakening connection with the subconscious, and the *Dynamic* phase moves us away from the intuitive world back to the rational, structured, outward focused thought processes of everyday awareness.

Like the *Creative* phase, it's a phase of transition where our physical energies and our orientation to the world change. Whereas the *Creative* phase is a time of decreasing physical energies and an increasing orientation towards the subconscious world, the *Dynamic* phase is one of increasing physical energy and an increasing orientation to the outer world. Both phases have a strong emphasis on ego and willpower and on what we want and need, and we can experience strong feelings of frustration when things don't meet our expectations. In particular in the *Dynamic* phase, this can be due to other people simply not keeping up with us as we burst with ideas, energy and schemes!

The subconscious can still impact disruptively on the *Dynamic* phase if we haven't allocated the required space and time to work with it in the *Creative* or *Reflective* phases. To give an example; this month I have been doing a lot of mental work, and now that I have moved into the *Dynamic* phase I'm pushing even harder to get reports written, projects structured and designed, and to catch up with things which have slipped down the priority list. This is all great *Dynamic* phase activity, but I'm also experiencing frustration and stress. Why? Because I didn't touch base with my deep inner needs during my *Creative* and *Reflective* phases.

The remedy is for me to allocate some rest time to give my subconscious feelings and needs the attention and validation they require. This can be more difficult to do in the *Dynamic* phase than in the other two phases, and I should have taken my own advice and done it at the Optimum Time.

We can also experience a reduction in emotional sensitivity or vulnerability in the *Dynamic* phase, making it the Optimum Time to have 'difficult' discussions such as making a complaint, standing up for our rights, putting our point across and asserting ourselves. However, this can mean that we appear to lack empathy, making it better to leave emotionally-based relationship discussions, such as supporting work colleagues or family and friends, until the more empathic *Expressive* phase.

The change from *Reflective* to *Dynamic* phase can vary from month to month. However, when we wake up feeling more confident and mentally sharp, and more motivated and enthusiastic, it's a good indicator that we have entered the *Dynamic* phase.

New month, new start

The *Dynamic* phase is a life-coaching dream! It's the Optimum Time for working out what we're going to do next in our lives, to understand which goals we will tackle this month, and to start detailing the milestone actions to make them happen.

Our high levels of self-confidence and enthusiasm at this time make motivation for starting new things, taking action, and stepping outside our 'comfort zone' really easy. We also naturally believe our positive self-talk, just as we naturally believed our negative self talk in the *Creative* phase, so it's the ideal time to use affirmations to fire up and guide our motivation.

The *Dynamic* phase is very much centered on **us**; our dreams, our needs and our wants, and we can come across as being very self-focused, goal-orientated, and lacking in compassion and patience. If we think about our energies in terms of the hormonal side of the menstrual cycle, this phase is very understandable. The *Dynamic* phase is the time before an egg is released, so we're less likely to get pregnant. Nature provides us with this unique space and set of abilities and energies to take action on our own personal dreams and to empower our individuality.

> **Nature provides us with the opportunity to create our personal goals and the optimum abilities to make them happen.**

Some women find it difficult to use the energy of the *Dynamic* phase because they feel uncomfortable at putting their needs before others'. They can view the natural approach of this phase as 'un-motherly' or unfeminine. However, this phase can be such a great Optimum Time for achievement, success, and moving forwards that many women experience the opposite feeling – that the phase doesn't last long enough!

The *Dynamic* phase gives us the opportunity to experience a more masculine energy and perception which, in the modern achievement and success-orientated business world, can be a huge advantage. If, however, we try to over-ride our other phases we lose out not only on some amazing abilities and opportunities for growth, but more importantly on the feelings of completeness, fulfillment and well-being generated by living in tune with each of our phases.

The *Dynamic* phase is the 'starting gun' going off, and if we stay in this phase we will never develop the stamina or commitment for the long distance run. When we use this phase as the starting point for new actions and projects, and support it with the nurturing of the *Expressive* phase, the creativity of the *Creative* phase, and the reviewing ability of the *Reflective* phase, we become empowered not only to make change but to fulfill seemingly unattainable long-term goals and heartfelt desires.

Dynamic phase positive self-talk

The *Dynamic* phase arrives with a strong belief in the positive. We are not only optimistic about the future but we also have a strong belief in ourselves. We naturally believe that we can do it, whatever 'it' may be!

In the chapter on the *Creative* phase we saw that positive affirmations – positive statements we make to change our thought processes – don't work because our responsive 'puppy mind' goes out and collects all the evidence for them not being true. In the *Dynamic* phase, however, it's not a case of needing evidence; we already feel deep down that it really is true.

So why use positive affirmations in this phase? The brain works on repetitive processes to build neural connections, and the more neural connections we make the more we are physically hot-wired to think and behave in a certain way. Repeating a beneficial statement about ourselves during the phase in which we naturally believe it helps us to fix the thought and accompanying emotions in our mindset.

Doing this creates a valuable tool to help carry positive emotions through into the more challenging *Creative* and *Reflective* phases.

If we work with affirmations throughout the *Dynamic* and *Expressive* phases, and work on acknowledging and releasing any underlying resistance in the subconscious during the *Creative* and *Reflective* phases, we have a powerful method to make deep and long-lasting changes. There are many books giving guidelines on using positive affirmations, but the simplest form is to create a short statement, in the present tense, about something we wish to have, be, experience or achieve. The statement is then either written down or stated out loud for a number of repetitions several times a day. See Day 11 of the Optimized Woman Daily Plan on creating a positive affirmation. Some of us may have already used affirmations without any perceived effect. As with any self-development method, it may be that the technique was not suited to the cycle phase when practiced.

The enthusiastic tendency of the *Dynamic* phase means we tend to over-emphasize and over-create affirmations to fit in with all the multiple goals and projects being developed. They can also become very long statements to cover everything! Often when these multiple affirmations are taken into the *Expressive* phase they will change naturally. We become more comfortable with simpler affirmations and will often reduce the number down to one or two core statements. We may also need to change the wording slightly in order to respond to them emotionally (see Day 14 of the Optimized Woman Daily Plan).

In the following month's *Dynamic* phase we may once again develop many more affirmations, but the most powerful ones will be the core statements which we repeat month after month.

Empowered anchoring

Another self-development method which benefits from being set up during the *Dynamic* phase and reinforced in the *Expressive* phase is a Neuro-Linguistic Programming (NLP) technique called 'anchoring'. This technique involves reliving or imagining a situation which generates positive feelings, and uses a physical trigger such as pressing two fingers together, to 'anchor' these feelings in our mindset. At a later date when we want to change our thoughts and feelings and recreate the ones we setup in the anchoring we simply enact the physical trigger.

In the *Dynamic* phase we are much more able to believe in positive imaginings and so the images and feelings we generate are stronger and appear more real, enhancing the anchoring technique.

During the *Creative* or *Reflective* phases, when we may want to encourage more positive thoughts and beliefs, we can use our trigger to reconnect and experience more optimistic feelings. Anchoring should not be used to try and fix these phases or to over-ride any negative thoughts or emotions. Remember that issues arise in our consciousness during the *Creative* and *Reflective* phases to be acknowledged and released as part of our way of supporting and maintaining our well-being and mental and emotional health. Using anchoring during these phases can help us to detach from emotionally committing to any negative thoughts and feelings, giving us the distance needed to acknowledge and work with them, and adding a bit more stability to our interaction with everyday life.

The Dynamic phase mind

Achievement, success and results are extremely important in the *Dynamic* phase. We not only feel the need for new projects to plan and structure for future successes, but we also need to achieve results right here, right now. Because we have the drive to take action and to achieve results quickly we can become very demanding, and when things don't develop – or people don't respond – quickly enough, we can experience intolerance, impatience and the frustration of feeling blocked.

For this reason we need to work on a number of different projects and goals at the same time, so that we can switch our attention and enthusiasm between them as and when they become blocked. We can then maintain the on-going sense of achievement necessary for our well-being in this phase, and juggling these additional projects is easy as our mental and multi-tasking skills are heightened.

These skills also mean that the *Dynamic* phase is the Optimum Time to catch up – not only on jobs we set aside in the Reflective phase but also on those lower priority jobs that never seem to reach the top of the 'to do' list.

The *Creative* phase can work hand-in-hand with the *Dynamic* phase by giving us the opportunity to clear the 'to do' list of items which are not important enough to carry forward into the new month and to provide ourselves with a prioritized list of urgent and important actions for the *Dynamic* phase.

The *Dynamic* phase is also the time to look realistically on what we have or haven't achieved to date. Identifying and acknowledging lack of success in this phase can be a powerful motivator to 'show them' rather than providing the evidence to prove what a failure we are, as is more likely in the *Creative* phase.

The greater memory recall in the *Dynamic* phase and an increase in our ability to process new information makes it the Optimum Time to research topics and details, learn new skills and information, go on courses, study self-development, catch up on background reading, work out how to implement new structures or software programs, explore how something works, read through legal or financial small print – the list is endless.

Our enhanced intellect and reasoning skills make us less emotionally sensitive and vulnerable and more able to view situations pragmatically, and empowers us to contemplate situations which could upset or frighten us in the other phases.

We have the strength not only to face these situations but also to analyze them and decide on and take appropriate action. This is the time to take a practical look at how the decisions we made in the *Creative* phase and committed to in the *Reflective* phase will impact on our life and the people around us. We are now more able to think logically through any consequences and to structure contingency plans.

This logical thinking ability also enables us to take a level-headed look at our work and at the future. We are more able to entertain thoughts of making radical changes, research necessary background information, weigh the consequences and risks, and create both short and long term strategies.

With our positive persona and self belief this is the Optimum Time for career advancement, taking steps to change careers, writing CVs and going to job interviews!

Planning the life you want

One of the keys to the Optimized Woman Daily Plan is planning, and it's in the *Dynamic* phase that we can really put this into action. We can use our powers of mental concentration to break down goals and task lists into manageable actions and timescales. We can plan for long-term projects, the month ahead or simply the day's action.

> "Will definitely now do future planning and organizing during the *Dynamic* and *Expressive* phases." Melanie, Teacher, UK.

Being aware of our cycle dates and our Optimum Times and their associated skills helps us to assess whether our planned tasks are in tune with our cycle, and we can use our *Dynamic* phase logical problem-solving abilities to structure activities or contingencies to coincide with them.

Where the *Dynamic* phase really has greatest impact is in planning long-term goals. Our cycles are a natural method of life-coaching ourselves, and it's in the *Dynamic* phase that we start planning our long-term goals and their associated action plans for the month ahead.

The classic life-coaching approach is to decide on an overall goal and a required achievement date, and then to create an action plan of smaller goals with target dates. Review dates are also set to help us keep a check on what we have achieved, what we haven't been able to achieve, and whether new opportunities have turned up which may influence our final goal.

One of the most frequent blocks to getting started is not knowing what it is that we really want to do, have or be. For years a friend said that he wanted to be able to play the guitar. When I suggested lessons, he would say that he didn't want to learn to play the guitar, he just wanted to be able to play it! Recently I said to him that I didn't believe he actually wanted to play the guitar, but rather I felt he just 'wished' he could play. If he really wanted to play, it wouldn't matter how many lessons it took, he would just be focused on his goal of playing. After a few days he came back to me saying he had decided to book his first lesson!

The difference between something we wish for and something we want is that we are willing to take action towards getting something we want.

We can use our cycles to find out what's important to us and what we want to do with our lives, and to help us to define our goals. We can use the *Dynamic* phase to research some initial ideas, the *Expressive* phase to talk things through with people around us, the *Creative* phase to ask our subconscious to help us feel and understand what it is we want from our lives, and then use the *Reflective* phase to internally process everything so that when we start the next *Dynamic* phase we are committed to the first steps towards changing our life.

Having chosen a long-term goal, the *Dynamic* phase becomes the phase to analyze the actions needed to achieve it and to plan the smaller tasks and their timescales. There can be a tendency in the *Dynamic* phase to go into too much detail, and we can create an overwhelming list of things 'to do'. Never look at it in the *Creative* phase! However, we can divide our main goal into a number of sub goals and then take just one of these and subdivide it into smaller actions for the month ahead. Looking through these smaller actions, our diaries, and our cycle dates, we can determine the Optimum Times to take these actions.

If during the previous month something has changed which impacts on our main goal, we can also use the *Dynamic* phase to reassess our long-term strategies and make changes to it. Long-term goals are not set in stone. Very often once we start traveling towards our goal new and amazing opportunities and situations can appear, seemingly out of the blue. The *Dynamic* phase is the Optimum Time to calculate what we need to change in order to take advantage of these new opportunities.

Dynamic phase Optimum Time

The *Dynamic* phase offers us new energies and enhanced abilities and skills, and to make sure that we use the phase productively we need to create strategies to make sure we don't miss them.

So what are these abilities, how can we make best use of this amazing phase, and what do we need to watch out for? Reading this section during the *Dynamic* phase may give you more ideas!

Dynamic phase abilities:

- Ability to itemize and prioritize.
- Creating structure and systems.
- Analysis and learning.
- Starting new projects.
- Enthusiasm and self-motivation.
- Confidence and positive thinking.
- Idealism.
- Independence and self-reliance.
- Inner drive to battle all challenges.
- Risk-taking.
- Concentration and memory recall.
- Championing others.
- Standing up for what is right.
- Logical problem solving and reasoning.
- Starting new projects.
- Structured learning, thinking and planning.
- Decision making.
- Excellent mental abilities.

What doesn't work so well in the Dynamic phase:

- Supporting others at an emotional level.
- Empathic understanding.
- Joint projects, working at another's pace.
- Abstract creativity and ideas.
- Going with the flow.
- Inactivity or lack of achievement.
- Giving power and responsibility to others.

- Team work.

Things to watch out for in the Dynamic phase:
- Frustration and annoyance when others don't keep up.
- Frustration due to lack of mental stimulus.
- Frustration due to lack of action, results or forward movement.
- More likely to make decisions and take risks without consulting others.
- Being too much 'in your head'.
- Starting something prematurely due to over-enthusiasm.
- Believing you are right in everything.
- Lack of patience and emotional understanding.
- Trying to fix everything and everyone at once.
- Being sociable but focused on self needs.
- Appearing cold and insensitive.
- Being seen to force, dictate or bully due to frustration.

Dynamic phase strategies:
Physical
- Restart the diet or fitness regime.
- Take regular exercise to burn off any excess energy.
- Physically challenge yourself with higher targets.
- Challenge yourself mentally and physically by learning a new physical activity.
- Start healthy eating.
- Quit smoking or break other habits.
- Alter routines.
- Take less sleep.
- Get outside more.
- Stimulate mind and body together.
- Start a class such as dance, step or anything aerobic.

Emotional
- Book evenings out socializing.

- Have fun reclaiming the outside world with trips, parties and events.
- Believe all the positive thoughts you have about yourself.
- Really enjoy catching up and all the things you can achieve.
- Enjoy starting new projects.
- Start learning new self-development techniques and allocating them to your phases.
- Avoid deep heart-to-heart conversations until the *Expressive* phase.
- Be aware of when you may be emotionally bullying others.
- Avoid feeling that this is the real 'you'.
- Accept that this phase will pass, so make the most of it!

Work

- Catch up on all the projects, tasks and jobs, put aside during the *Reflective* phase.
- Multi-task to get more done.
- Make contact with people again after the Reflective phase hibernation.
- Learn something new; go on a course or get that software manual out!
- Learn something complex; you may surprise yourself on what you can understand and retain in this phase.
- Analyze reports and figures, do calculations.
- Create reports, graphs, structures and rationales.
- Create strategic and tactical plans.
- Investigate details, break things down to their smallest elements.
- Take the overview approach, plan long-term.
- Assert points of view, ideas and expertise.
- Fight for what you think is right
- Take on difficult conversations requiring a detached approach e.g. customer complaints.
- Give co-workers time to catch up, or leave their input until the *Expressive* phase when team working is easier.

- Try not to appear too demanding or dictatorial in communications.
- Where possible, try to work on projects alone; this enables you to work at our own pace.
- Negotiate or mediate where an analytical, observer viewpoint is required.
- Pitch ideas, but ideally leave face-to-face meetings until the Expressive phase.
- Choose a couple of projects as a release for feelings of enthusiasm and motivation.
- Make doing pleasurable things outside of work as high a priority as work itself.
- Use feelings of enthusiasm to motivate co-workers rather than bully them.
- Set up time management systems to support later phases.
- Plan meetings, tasks and deadlines to support the other phases and to make use of their enhanced abilities for that Optimum Time.

Goal fulfillment:

- Create action plans for the month ahead.
- Start taking action immediately on multiple tasks.
- Learn new skills and approaches which can help with success and goal achievement.
- Compare approaches and actions with other people's progress and successes, and learn from them.
- Use affirmations to program your mind towards self-confidence and success for the rest of the month.
- Use positive affirmations to support your goals.
- Formalize long term goals and plans.
- Research information to support actions and plans.
- Look for analytical and review data in the goal area.
- Follow the money; work on financial plans and projections.
- Plan and take immediate action on any healthy eating,

dieting or fitness regimes linked to goals.

- Push forward on 'bad habit' goals by reducing a negative aspect or increasing a positive aspect.

The challenge:

- To keep our feet on the ground.
- To use enthusiasm to motivate rather than bully.
- To accept that everything doesn't happen as quickly as we'd like.
- To acknowledge the feelings and input of others.

Your ideas for Dynamic phase activities:

Chapter 7

Working with the Optimum Time of the Expressive phase

The Ovulation phase may be a subtle phase for some women to recognize because the change in energies and perception can develop gradually. However, some of us may be aware of a number of physical changes that can happen with the release of the egg, and these help remind us to look at our abilities and attitude and acknowledge that we are in our *Expressive* phase.

One reason why the phase can be difficult to identify is that many of us see the abilities and attitude of this phase to be the epitome of womanhood and how we feel we should be all the time. It's often experienced as the 'real me', while two of the other three phases are viewed as dysfunctional.

The *Expressive* phase is a wonderful phase, with feelings of joy and happiness, creativity and self-expression, confidence and fulfillment, altruism and love. It is a feeling-orientated phase but, unlike the more introspective feelings experienced during the *Creative* phase, these feelings are naturally positive and are linked to relationships and to connecting with and creating the world around us.

> "(*Expressive phase*) A good time for creative work such as story writing, planning and writing reports. Lesson planning is also easier as the ideas come more steadily." Melanie, Teacher, UK.

Whatever attitude we bring to this phase, whether it's the relief of returning to ourselves, joy at touching base with our femininity, comfort or discomfort at experiencing 'traditional' female energies, or the frustration as the drive of the *Dynamic* phase fades, it offers us powerful skills and abilities for enhancing both our personal and working lives.

Expressive phase overview

The *Expressive* phase abilities and skills develop around the time of ovulation and are usually experienced a few days before and a few days afterwards. Like the *Reflective* phase, the *Expressive* phase is a pivot time in our cycle, characterized by a weakening of the driving force of the ego.

Where the *Reflective* phase is a time of inner withdrawal and renewal, the Expressive phase is a time for us to reach out and express ourselves and our energies into the world. Our ego seems to give way to a more altruistic focus where our wants, desires and goals become less important to us and we become more empathic and aware of the needs around us. We know the *Expressive* phase is ending when we experience the increasingly driven energies of the *Creative* phase and become more self-orientated and less tolerant!

During the Expressive phase, work colleagues' and customers' needs and feelings have a higher priority than our own projects. We are also more willing to 'go with the flow' and to allow things to develop in their own time. We are more likely to nurture projects, to create the right environment for them and the people involved to develop in an organic way, than to be the visionary powerhouse forcing everyone to follow our direction.

The emotional level-headedness of the *Dynamic* phase develops into emotional strength in the *Expressive* phase. Here it combines with patience and acceptance, enabling us to ask for and validate other people's viewpoints and input. We find ourselves less sensitive to criticism and more able to understand the feelings and motivation behind people's words or actions. Our natural caring attitude and our ability to listen and communicate well means that this is the Optimum Time for supporting both projects and people through heart-to-heart meetings, team building, mediating compromises, negotiating win-win deals and networking to create new business and work contacts as well as friendships.

Throughout the *Expressive* phase, our sense of personal well-being is directly related to expressing our feelings of love, appreciation, gratitude and caring. Caring for our family and socializing with friends is a big part of supporting ourselves during this phase. Our inner strength also means we can be involved in people's lives without becoming overwhelmed by their needs, something we can easily experience in the *Creative* phase. When we think about this phase from nature's point of view, nature is preparing us to become mothers; to care about a child and to create the social connections through which our child and ourselves are supported by others.

The *Expressive* phase is our Optimum Time to step out into the world to make the connections we need to succeed in our careers and goals, and our natural approach can be very 'feminine'.

In the *Dynamic* phase we can tend to gravitate towards men for a more masculine approach to making things happen, while in the *Expressive* phase we may be drawn towards a more relationship-based approach. We may find that we behave very differently towards male and female colleagues during this time, and that men subconsciously react to the 'femininity' of this phase. Depending on our views we can use this knowledge to our advantage, or we can ignore it or feel uncomfortable about it.

In the *Expressive* phase we have the inner emotional strength and the extrovert tendencies to express who we are and the fantastic skills and abilities we have to offer! When we use the full potential of this phase we can make a positive impact on our careers and goals, and on our families and friendships.

The Expressive phase creativity

The menstrual cycle is a cycle of female creative energy expressed in all its forms. Unfortunately we often have difficulties in understanding exactly what being creative means and how it applies to what we do in everyday life.

If we ask ourselves 'Are we creative?' the answer is very often 'no' because we tend to think of creativity as painting a master-piece or writing an orchestral symphony or a literary tome. Creativity however has a much wider range of forms than these, and is an active part of every woman's cycle and life.

Creativity is the action rather than the outcome. It's expressed in inspiration, the leap in understanding, problem–solving, blue sky thinking, planning and in imagining. It is found in adver-tising, teaching, presenting, managing and in team-building. It appears in 'creating' structure, balance and harmony, co-worker relationships, public relations and customer service, effective communi-cation and in creating order out of chaos.

As well as all this, creativity is found in the areas we more normally tend to

> "I love the *Expressive* phase. I feel very caring and have the patience to sit and do crafts for friends and family... making things feels as though I am expressing my thoughts and feelings into the world." Jo, Receptionist, Australia.

associate with the word; art and design, writing and music, dance and singing, acting and performance, as well as in those more associated with 'feminine' tasks such as caring and nurturing, nursing and healing, cooking and sewing, gardening, homemaking and bringing up children.

In fact all of the above are 'feminine' creative abilities; we just have Optimum Times during the month for expressing our creative energies in particular ways.

> **When we redefine our view of 'creativity' the whole cycle becomes a vibrant and exciting creative opportunity.**

The *Expressive* phase is the Optimum Time for the more traditionally 'female' creative abilities. No, this doesn't mean we have to go out and bake cakes or knit booties, although this can be a very good way to support our own well-being during this phase. What it does mean is that we have some exciting people management and communication skills, as well as intrinsic practical application and development capabilities, plus a flair for teaching and mediation. On top of all of this we also have a whole load of emotional strength.

The 'motherly' Expressive phase and the extended family

During the *Expressive* phase, the people we work with can become an extended part of the group of people we care about (our 'family') and we can use our enhanced nurturing skills to create better and deeper relationships and communication.

The reduced drive of the ego and the heightened ability to empathize makes this the Optimum Time to talk to people. As we are less likely to get upset or to read perceived criticism into our interactions with other people, we can use this time to find out how co-workers really feel about a project or working conditions and how customers experience our service. We are also more willing to spend time with people, so this is the ideal opportunity to re-establish relationships with family, friends and work colleagues who may have felt neglected during the *Reflective* and *Dynamic* phases.

In the *Expressive* phase we are also more able to actively listen and to validate the views of others so we can proactively ask for ideas and suggestions without feeling any threat to our position. We can effectively use this phase for employee job appraisals as we are more able to communicate appreciation and interest in their concerns, and to offer practical support in their role and work. We can still point out faults and issues, but we will be doing it in a more empathic and understanding way, giving them the motivation to put things right and the emotional support to believe that they can do it.

For team leaders this is the Optimum Time for reinforcing the team relationship by reviewing each member's viewpoint, settling conflicts, creating support for workflows, and making each person feel that their contribution to the team is appreciated and valued. This also applies to family 'teams'.

In essence, the *Expressive* phase enables us to create continuing, supportive and mutually beneficial relationships. We can use this ability not only to support project teams but also to cultivate and maintain our own expanded 'team' of people who support us in our work. This expanded group includes everyone from the technical help guy, the secretary, the boss, co-workers, suppliers and service providers to our work mentor, business advisor or life coach, counselor, best friend, partner and family members.

The *Expressive* phase provides us with the ability to strengthen the relationships that strengthen us, and it also gives us the ability to communicate in such a way as to get the best from these relationships. We have the sociability and energy to interact with people directly and to give them our attention to show that their relationship and support is important to us. In return, we get people who can be sounding boards for ideas or problems, people who can help with extra workload or responsibilities, people who have the power to make our lives a bit easier, and people who may have the connections to help advance us in our career or goals. We get people who support us no matter what we do, who believe in our abilities, and who will encourage and motivate us when the going gets tough.

The phase to shine and get what you want!

The *Expressive* phase not only brings superior communication skills and inner strength but also the awareness and patience to get what you want by gently persuading people.

In the *Dynamic* phase we may stride into the boss's office and state that we want a pay rise and here is a list of reasons why we deserve it. In the *Expressive* phase we are more likely to orchestrate a seemingly casual encounter with the boss and lead the conversation round to highlighting the benefits of our work, and planting the seed idea of a pay rise. As this is an Optimum Time for nurturing, we can then nurture this pay rise idea over a few days, helping the boss to think it is his or her own.

During this phase we are much more able to take a tactical approach to getting what we want, and we have the patience and awareness to help people come round to our idea or viewpoint. So am I saying that this is the Optimum Time for manipulating people? Yes!

> **The Expressive phase is the Optimum Time to encourage, guide, persuade, influence and manipulate.**

This may seem calculating; however, within the *Expressive* phase where feelings and altruism are important to us our manipulation of people comes from a heartfelt caring, guiding and leading approach.

We are also more likely to compromise due to understanding and appreciating the other person's point of view or circumstances, but we are also more able to put across our own viewpoint and have the confidence to negotiate from a position of self-worth and inner strength.

We are like a patient mother trying to teach and persuade her child that the apple is a better choice than the candy bar.

We are also more emotionally immune from any anger or backlash our approach may have, and so are more likely to stay with the situation and look for a positive resolution rather than backing down, walking away or becoming confrontational.

The *Expressive* phase is the best Optimum Time to sell ourselves, our work and our product or service. We have the confidence and communication skills to productively 'cold call', network, present meetings and attend events, which ultimately become opportunities for advancement and success. The introduction at a conference could lead to being head-hunted, the afternoon of cold-calling could lead to a large account, our ringing a number of suppliers could bring cost cuts, and the timely telephone call could lead to the job of our dreams. This is also the time to touch base with clients or customers and suggest new products or services, to ask for feedback, and to listen to what they want or anticipate needing. Relationships are always two-way, so this is also a great time to highlight to others how we are helping them. We can take clients out and do some schmoozing to help people to see not only our company's good points but also our own.

The Expressive phase peacemaker

One of the most powerful characteristics of the *Expressive* phase is the reduction in ego-fuelled drive and subconscious generated fears and anxieties. This means that we are able to step back emotionally from aggressive people and conflict situations and deal with them from an impartial and open standpoint. We have the awareness, the understanding and the communication skills needed to defuse aggression in other people, as well as the ability to see both sides of a situation and to empathize with conflicting parties. This gives us the ability to be productive mediators and arbitrators.

Just as we can get the best from a team in this Optimum Time, we can also get the best from everyone in meetings, even those people with conflicting viewpoints and needs. Add to this our ability to create compromise, and we can turn potentially destructive meetings into productive ones.

How we handle a conflict meeting can be different depending on our phase. In the *Reflective* phase we could be more likely to pull away and not get involved, in the *Dynamic* phase we may try logic and focus to solve the problem but find we are seen as cold and dictatorial, and in the *Creative* phase we may have the flash of inspiration to create the ultimate solution but have no one commit because they are too busy fighting for territory.

The *Expressive* phase approach may simply be one of re-creating positive relationships between the conflicting parties so that insight, logic and inspiration can be called into play at a later date and be well received by both parties.

In the *Expressive* phase we're not looking for the quick fix; instead we are willing to **take the long term solution, to nurture something to grow into what we want and to make sure that we take everyone with us on the journey**.

Jumping in puddles!

The *Expressive* phase is also about having fun and celebrating life. We can experience heightened feelings of gratitude during this phase, and it's our enjoyment of what we have that makes us feel happy and want to celebrate. Many self-development books teach that to be happy we need to feel more appreciation for what we have rather than always striving for the next material, work-related, personal or relationship goal. The *Expressive* phase naturally gives us this appreciative attitude.

As with all the other phases, if we miss interacting with our Optimum Time we lose a wonderful opportunity to put our cyclic skills and abilities to positive use.

Ignoring the *Expressive* phase Optimum Time means we pass over the potential to feel deep gratitude, joy and happiness and the opportunity to express these feelings in two wonderful ways; giving and play.

The appreciation we have for who we are and what we have naturally expresses itself in an altruistic desire to give. In the work environment it can manifest as giving extra time to clients and customers, helping co-workers with their tasks, listening or being with someone, or simply getting someone a coffee! Fulfillment comes not only from feeling happy but also from sharing.

We can also express our happiness and joy of who we are and our environment through play. So our day job is being a CEO in a multi-billion dollar corporate empire… but when was the last time we celebrated our joy of life by jumping in puddles? Play is an action which is fun, sensual, creative yet pointless (apart from the fact that it is fun) and unproductive.

Many of the traditionally 'feminine' creative expressions fit themselves into this concept of play during the *Expressive* phase. It's the knitting which is important not the scarf, the act of touching the earth or the plant which is important not the garden, the cooking which is important not the cake (unless of course it's chocolate cake!).

Play can also be meditative; we can lose our thinking and worrying self in the fun of the activity. It's interesting that although the *Expressive* and *Reflective* phases are opposite each other in the cycle, they are both phases of meditation – 'active' meditation in the *Expressive* phase and 'stillness' meditation in the *Reflective*.

Losing ourselves in play helps us to reconnect with who we truly are underneath the expectations we and other people have about ourselves, and this makes it a powerful tool for stress relief. The effect of play is more powerful during this phase if it is sensual and creative, and truly without a purpose other than itself.

Making time to play during the *Expressive* phase can help us stay happy, grounded and stress-free, which in turn helps us to be better at our work and better at nurturing and supporting the important relationships in our life.

It's clear to see why many women wish to stay in this phase all the time; they feel good about themselves, experience deep levels of happiness and well-being, feel loving and giving towards others, and feel emotionally strong, patient and capable. But this phase comes because of the phases which precede and follow it. Without the phases which allow the ego to explore and drive its wants and needs, we wouldn't have the rounded personality which could offer altruistic support for all. Without the withdrawal into the depths of ourselves in the *Reflective* phase, there would be no renewal to allow us to shine in the *Expressive* phase. Without the drive and assertiveness of the dynamic phases, we would not be able to fight the battles to create a better world.

> **Our strength and power lie not in one phase but in the flow of changing phases, each supporting the other and creating the women we are.**

Being our own cheerleader

The *Expressive* phase is also an important time for us to connect with and build our confidence and self-esteem. So often we are continually striving for the next goal or trying to clear the list of 'things to do' that we never give time to appreciate our successes. The more stressed the situation, the closer the deadlines, the longer the list of tasks, the less and less likely we are to appreciate what we have achieved and the more our focus tends to be on simply managing. Any concept of feeling gratitude and success seems unreachable. However, it is the experience of feeling successful which helps us to build self-confidence and to have a deep inner knowing that we are strong enough and self-contained enough not only to achieve what we want, but also to manage difficult situations with calm and strength.

Self-confidence comes from knowing who we are and what we can do, and this in turn comes from emotionally experiencing our achievements and successes. When we don't give ourselves time to experience the positive emotions of success, we can find ourselves looking to other people or external situations to generate them for us.

The *Expressive* phase is the Optimum Time to build our feelings of success, confidence and achievement into our sense of who we are. We can do this easily because appreciation is a natural part of how we think in this phase.

Experiencing success emotions establishes a base-line of self-confidence and self-worth which runs throughout the month, and the more we feel our successes the higher this baseline will grow.

Notice that I've been talking about 'feelings'. During the *Expressive* phase our feelings are the most important way that we express and interact with the world around us. To build our self-confidence we need to feel our success. We can use our intellect to review the month and see what we have achieved, but we also need to awaken the emotion of success and achievement. The abilities of the *Expressive* phase make this easier now than at any other time of the month.

When we ignore the *Expressive* phase and don't give ourselves time to emotionally feel our successes we are losing out on the greatest cheerleader we could have; ourselves! We miss an opportunity to build success into our core emotional belief and to encourage positive self-esteem and an attitude of self-confidence.

Every month we miss this amazing opportunity.

As the *Expressive* phase ends, we can experience a decline in our extroverted energies and a build-up of the more emotionally sensitive and inspirational experiences of the *Creative* phase. Now things start to get really exciting, so hold on tight as once again we ride the creative and inspirational rollercoaster.

Expressive phase Optimum Time

The *Expressive* phase presents us with a wide range of abilities and skills which we can use effectively in our personal and working life. Try being aware of the different abilities listed below, and try applying them in the suggested actions. Use the space provided to add your own ideas for *Expressive* phase activities.

Abilities:
- Empathy and an altruistic outlook.
- Creating connections and supportive relationships.
- Effective communication and people skills.
- Feelings-orientated.
- Flexible, able to compromise, arbitrate and negotiate.
- Enjoyment of life, happiness and playfulness.
- Patience and gentleness.
- Creating support.
- Ability to be aware of and understand other people's needs.
- To persuade, guide, teach, and lead.
- To sacrifice own needs and wants.
- Active listening and validation.
- Feeling and expressing gratitude and appreciation.
- Gentleness, nurturing and caring.
- Reading faces and body language.
- Understanding people's feelings and motivation.
- Generosity and giving.
- Geniality and charm.

- Ability to feel success.
- Flexibility to change your routine to fit in with others.
- Ability to accept people and situations as they are.
- Nest building and home-making.
- Everyday practical care for people and surroundings.

What doesn't work:

- Long term self-sacrifices, as the impulse may be generated by the phase but go against your deeper needs. Run the idea through your Creative and Reflective phases first.
- Expecting a go-getting, aggressive dynamic attitude.
- Blue-sky thinking.
- Spending time away from home; the home can be important to well-being in this phase.
- Trying to be masculine.
- Motivation for material goals.
- Analyzing detail.
- Logical thinking.
- Working overtime or bringing work home.
- Doing things on your own.

Things to watch out for:

- Signing up for too much extra work or responsibilities to help others.
- People taking advantage of you; you can be too generous.
- Not meeting your own needs, leading to frustration.
- No time for yourself.
- Guilt if you are not doing things for others.
- Guilt at not being able to solve all the world's problems.
- Self worth being dependent on how other people see and react to you.
- Giving away too much in meetings.
- Not acting quickly.
- Going with the flow can negate your needs and

preferences.
- Smaller personal body space and a willingness to touch.
- Time spent supporting or networking can be interpreted as unproductive.
- Lack of drive can be seen as lack of interest and commitment.
- Expecting to be like this all the time.

Strategies:

Physical
- Enjoy your sociability and visit friends and family.
- Go to events and classes to make new friends and relationships.
- Make time for doing the things you enjoy.
- Get out into nature.
- Indulge your senses and enjoy them!
- Physically touch people (when and where appropriate!)
- Exercise, walk, dance, and have fun with your body.
- Eat your favorite foods, consciously savor and enjoy every bite.
- Put your creativity into action, find a playful pastime.
- Enjoy your successes at the gym.

Emotional
- Have heart-to-heart conversations.
- Give counseling to others.
- Broach difficult subjects.
- Do some charity or volunteer work.
- Spend more quality time with partner, family and friends.
- Support others, either through communications or actions.
- Look at how you can create better relationships with people and put any ideas into action.
- Give in when appropriate, but do not lose sight of your own needs.
- Have a family meeting to allow expression, arbitration and

problem solving.

- Give hugs.
- Tell people how much you appreciate them and how you feel about them.
- Give simple gifts to express gratitude.
- Do things which make you feel successful and feminine (buy that expensive designer dress you desire!)
- Set aside extra time to play with your children and partner.
- List your everyday successes and feel really good about them.
- Motivate yourself by seeing your tasks meeting other people's needs in some way.

Work

- Go to meetings, conferences, exhibitions, work groups and business club meetings to broaden your networking.
- Start casual conversations to create new contacts.
- Run team support meetings and facilitate free expression of views, ideas, complaints and issues.
- Focus your skills on any disputes and create compromise and solutions.
- Create 'chance meetings' to help mediate and negotiate conflicts.
- Mentor or help guide and support people.
- Run an 'open door' policy for this week, allowing anyone to pop in and air problems, ideas or issues.
- Do staff assessments.
- Identify people, projects and areas which need support to grow, maintain productivity or manage change.
- Take a nurturing approach to people and projects. Give them the freedom to run until they go off track or make mistakes and then actively guide them round to the right direction.
- Get out on to the 'shop floor' and talk face-to-face with staff, customers or suppliers.

- Offer to teach during this phase, as you have the communication skills.
- Present yourself as being approachable, helpful, fair and impartial.
- Create a campaign to sell yourself both within your company or organization and to clients and customers.
- Use this time to present your ideas and run a contact / network campaign to get them endorsed by others.
- Talk to people; give your attention and listen and motivate.
- Contact people who you think could help solve problems or support your projects. Ask for help where necessary; you won't mind refusal.
- Appreciate how much you do for people.
- Contact suppliers to thank them, and show appreciation to co-workers and staff.
- Find creative outlets you can do easily at work; perhaps doodle, write a poem or take some knitting to work!
- Appreciate how much you have learned and achieved in the past month.
- Feminize your work space, create a comfortable 'home' at work.
- Talk to you boss. Find out what he / she wants, how you can help and most importantly subtly show what a good worker you are.
- Make a conscious effort to connect with other women at work or in your industry / specialism.
- Use your communication skills to sell your ideas to people. Aim high.
- Identify people's underlying feelings and motivation and use this information to adapt your approach.
- Use this time to learn relational systems, and to review connections, workflow, reporting, and management guidelines.
- Share information with different departments, clients and

co-workers to develop new lines of communication.

Goal fulfillment:

- Target and contact people who may be able to help you meet your goal.
- Ask people for input on your ideas and approach.
- Ask for face-to-face meetings, as you will be better at communicating this way.
- Take your goals and look for connections that exist between them.
- Focus on your successes to date; reward yourself, because you are worth it!
- Practice presenting your ideas to people; develop a 17 second introduction.
- Evaluate the positive impact achieving your goal will have on others.
- Take time to appreciate your journey to your goal; what have you learned, how have you grown?
- Look at how you can persuade people to help you; is there a win-win solution?

The challenge:

- Not to surrender all your needs.
- To develop your self-worth without relying on other people.
- To accept that this phase will pass and not take on too many emotional demands and responsibilities.
- To give yourself time to play and enjoy life.
- To stay motivated towards personal material goals.

Your ideas for Expressive phase activities:

Chapter 8

Introduction to the daily plan

Before starting the Optimized Woman Daily Plan it is useful to understand the approach of the plan and the key tools for working with it. We'll also look at how to get started and a number of frequently asked questions.

The Optimized Woman Daily Plan

The Optimized Woman Daily Plan is the first self-development approach specifically designed for women based on the cyclic abilities inherent in the menstrual cycle. The plan succeeds where others fail by tying actions and techniques to the enhanced abilities experienced in four Optimum Times within the cycle.

The Optimized Woman Daily Plan is designed to create awareness of our cyclic nature, to help us to under-stand in more depth our unique experiences of each phase, and to discover life-enhancing ways of applying our knowledge and heightened abilities practically in our lives. By working through the plan we have the opportunity to discover each Optimum Time and use its empowering associated abilities to create

> Miranda Gray's 28 day plan has helped me build a greater respect, appreciation and understanding of my menstrual cycle. Before starting the plan I felt very disconnected from my cycle and saw menstruation as a burden. After starting the plan not only did it help to reconnect me to it, I started to see the power and beauty in understanding it. Tess, Human Resources, Canada.

impactful and dynamic life changes.

The plan offers:

- Information on the powerful experiences, potentials and opportunities intrinsic in each phase.
- Suggestions on how to best use the physical, mental and emotional energies and abilities of our Optimum Time.
- Practical daily actions for well-being, goal achievement and work progess.
- Ways to help us support our needs and enjoy the phase.
- Strategies to help when circumstances don't fit our Optimum Time.
- The flexibility to enable us to individualize the daily plan to create our own personal monthly plan for achieving our full potential.

Using the daily plan can radically change the way we view our abilities, enabling us to go beyond our perceived limitations. Our cycles become an empowering resource of amazing abilities and opportunities that we can apply to tasks and actively use to excel and to create the success and fulfillment we desire.

Daily actions

Each day in the plan consists of a daily focus, information on an aspect of the abilities of the Optimum Time, a well-being action, a goal achievement action, and a work enhancement action.

These daily actions are designed to help in the following areas:

1. Well-being: confidence and self esteem, creativity, lifestyle, relationships and acceptance, exploring what it means to be cyclic, and using the Optimum Times to enhance our sense of well-being.

2. Goal achievement: identifying our true goals, when and what type pf action to take, building motivation, and using our

Optimum Times to provide the necessary support to achieve our goals and dreams.

3. Work enhancement: utilizing our full potential, allocating tasks to Optimum Times, planning and strategies, working more effectively, empowering our work practice, and creating career opportunities.

We can either concentrate on a single type of daily action for one cycle or choose whichever action from the three fits in best with our day.

To start with, it's better to work with just one of the three activity types, for example only the goal achievement actions, for a whole cycle. This gives us the opportunity to really notice how our cycle influences this area of our life and how working with our Optimum Times releases our full potential and empowers us to make change and take impactful action.

To start, work on a single area for a whole cycle for maximum benefit.

Making the plan work for you

The Optimized Woman Daily Plan is a guide or a map of the cyclic changes experienced each month; however, the journey through the cycle is ours alone to take. To help us discover our Optimum Times and their mental, emotional and physical changes we need to take the journey with three basic provisions. Firstly we need to **compare the experiences** of each phase; secondly we need to **notice the activities we find easy**; and thirdly we need to **acknowledge that we change**.

Compare phases

To gain awareness of our changes we need to compare our abilities in different phases. To do this we can ask ourselves some questions:

'What tasks do I find easier, which abilities are more enhanced, and what is my natural approach to things?'

'Am I more emotionally responsive and empathic in some phases compared to others? When do I experience my heightened ability to be altruistic?'

'Does my creativity and problem-solving have peaks? When do I experience my enhanced creative abilities and how do I express them?'

'Can I understand and manage complex issues better in certain phases? When are my mental abilities sharpest and my multi-tasking ability strongest?'

'Am I better at expressing myself in different phases? When do I feel my ability to communicate is enhanced?'

'When am I most frustrated? What aspect of my phase am I over-riding?'

By noticing our changes and comparing how our abilities change from one Optimum Time to the next we will discover our own unique pattern of heightened skills and abilities.

While using the plan, many women like to keep a journal about their experiences and whether the daily actions suggested fit their abilities. However, in our busy working lives we don't always have the time to keep a journal, so at the end of each Optimum Time there is a quick summary sheet for recording experiences. Not only do these summaries help to identify our unique experiences of each Optimum Time, but at the end of a cycle they also help us to compare our abilities across all four Optimum Times more easily.

By keeping a record we uncover the types of heightened abilities we experience in which Optimum Times, and we can use this information to plan tasks for the month ahead to make sure that we make the best possible use of our enhanced abilities.

Notice what you can do

We are much more likely to notice what we can't do rather than what we can do' and this often creates a negative approach to our cycle and feelings of frustration and self-criticism. As one Optimum Time changes into the next we need to actively look for the gifts of the new phase and be inventive on how we use them.

Ask yourself 'What do I find easy and what can I do with this ability to excel, create change or achieve my goals?'

"When I am menstrual I feel more confident and more organised. I find structure and organization easier and am more assertive. These tasks are normally really difficult for me because of my Dyslexia and Dyspraxia." Pollyanne, Housing Management Officer, UK.

The answer may surprise you and open up new and exciting opportunities!

Acknowledge that you change

Once we acknowledge that our abilities change during our cycles we can stop fighting our cyclic nature and instead work with it to focus our Optimum Time energies on the things we want to create and achieve. So often we try to be constant throughout the month to meet our expectations of who we believe we are and what we should achieve. Our society and working environments also expect us to be constant in our abilities, putting even more pressure on us to always have the same level of skills and the same skill sets.

When we acknowledge that we change and work with our changes we release stress and create more feelings of well-being. We also enter a whole new and empowered way of viewing ourselves, our self-development, career and goals.

We are not going to change the business world or society overnight, but we can recognize that our cyclic changes give us the opportunity to achieve more and to shine!

Before starting the plan you may also find it useful to revisit the five keys to success in *Chapter 2*.

> **Once you have worked with the plan, the way you think about yourself and your life will change forever!**

Getting started

To start the Optimized Woman Daily Plan you can simply look at the page for the particular day of your cycle. Remember that day 1 is the first day of your menstruation.

The best day to start the plan is the first day of the *Dynamic* phase. As we've already seen, the *Dynamic* phase is the Optimum Time for starting new projects, so you may like to start the plan on day 7.

If you don't know the day you are currently on, make a rough guess. If the plan content for the day doesn't fit your experiences you can always go forward or backward through the plan to a day which seems to fit better.

> **The Optimum Time to start the plan is on day 7 of your cycle.**

Read through the text for the day and then choose the appropriate action depending on which of the three areas you wish to work on. Ideally, work through a whole cycle for each of the individual areas.

Once you have worked with the plan, the way you think about yourself and your life will change! Your relationship with your cycle will also change, and you will look forward to each phase in anticipation of the powerful tools and resources it has waiting for you. These tools have always been there; they've just been waiting for you to recognize them and put them to good use

---

If you want to get ahead – get a cycle!

Frequent questions about the Optimized Woman Daily Plan

1. My cycle is rarely regular but the plan is 28 days long; can I still use it?

Yes you can. With a longer or shorter cycle, your Optimum Times may change on different days to those mentioned in the plan. As you work through the daily plan, see if the suggested actions fit in well with your abilities and feelings; if not, look further forwards in the plan or go back a few days to find an action which seems to fit.

2. My abilities and cycle day number don't seem to fit your plan – does it mean that something is wrong with me?

No, nothing is wrong! Every woman's cycle is unique to her, and very often the experience of a cycle can change from month to month. It may well be that in your natural cycle your Creative phase is two weeks long rather than a week, or your Reflective phase could be only be three days long!

The idea of this book is to help you to **become aware of your own unique cycle and abilities** and to find practical ways of using these abilities at your Optimum Times. My advice is to experiment and use the plan as a way to discover your unique cycle.

If you find that your *Creative* phase is two weeks long, simply spend two days on each day action instead of one. If your *Reflective* phase is only three days long, simply start the *Dynamic* phase early. As you get to know your own unique cycle and its abilities you will begin to be more aware of when your changes occur and know how to take best advantage of your Optimum Times.

3. I am on the contraceptive pill / have had a hysterectomy. Can I still use the plan?

If you experience a hormonal cycle, whether artificial or natural, with or without a womb, there is no reason why you cannot use the plan. You may find that your experiences are different from those mentioned, but the plan will help you to become aware of your abilities and discover your Optimum Times. It will also give you some great practical ideas on how to use these abilities.

4. I am menopausal, is it worth me using the plan or is it too late?

No it's not too late, and in fact the plan is ideal for menopausal women. Obviously you won't be experiencing a regular cycle, but the plan can help you to recognize the changes in your abilities and suggest positive and practical ways of using these abilities when you have them. If your *Reflective* phase lasts for weeks, it can be a great gift to have this extra time to really look at your life and decide what is important and what you want to do. If your *Dynamic* phase lasts for months you have a wonderful opportunity to get things done and make things happen.

Use the plan and use this time in your life to create the future you want.

5. Why do you start the plan on day 7?

Day 7 is the start of the *Dynamic* phase when we experience increasing levels of physical and mental energy. It's the Optimum Time for starting new projects, and so the ideal time for starting the plan.

6. Can I start the plan if I don't know what day of the month I am currently on?

Yes you can. You can take a guess at where you are in your current cycle and see if the information and actions seem to fit in with your energies and abilities. If they don't correspond, look a few days forward or back in the plan to find a day that fits.

7. Are there really four phases in my cycle?

The answer to this is both yes and no.

The menstrual cycle is based around two events, ovulation and menstruation, and on the changes in hormones at and between these two events. The cycle is a complex flow of physical, mental and emotional experiences, which means that your natural expression and abilities gradually change throughout your cycle. For example, the beginning of your *Creative* phase will be a blend of *Creative* and *Expressive* phase attributes, while towards the end of the phase you're more likely to experience a blend of *Creative* and *Reflective* phase energies and attributes.

To help you identify what happens during the cycle, individual cycle days have been grouped into four phases of similar attributes, your Optimum Times. This makes it much easier for you to make comparisons across the cycle, and by comparing experiences you are able to realize that your abilities change naturally from week to week.

Using the four hormonal phases is a good place to start. However, if you go on to create the personal Cycle Dial outlined in *Chapter 10* you may well find that you can identify more than four distinct repeating phases within your own cycle.

8. Surely other things change my abilities and feelings as well as my cycle?

Yes, there are many things which can have an impact on your abilities and how you perceive the world. These can include illness, medication, lack of sleep, crossing time zones, drugs and alcohol, stress, love, and exercise to name a few!

For this reason it's useful to keep a record of your abilities and feelings for a few months so you can recognize your underlying pattern.

9. Can my young daughter use the plan?

There is no reason why you can't introduce the ideas of the plan to your daughter. In fact it's important that we share our experiences with the younger generation so that they develop their own understanding of their unique cyclic abilities.

10. How can a phase be *'creative'* when I feel creative throughout the month?

The menstrual cycle is a cycle of changing forms of creativity. You can create new actions in the pre-ovulation phase, relationships during ovulation, inspired ideas in the pre-menstrual phase and deep connections within yourself during menstruation.

The names chosen for the phases try to encapsulate the core pattern behind each phase. The *Creative* phase reflects the mind's strong ability in this phase to create reality through both negative thoughts and inspired insights and ideas, and the urge to create something physical even if it's only to create order in a messy room.

11. I am seeing a life-coach / business coach. Does the plan clash with what I am already doing with them?

No. The Optimized Woman Daily Plan fits in well with any sort of coaching as you usually determine your own goals, achievement deadlines and review dates, so you can align them with your

Optimum Times. You can share the concept of the plan with your coach, or you simply fit your action plan around your Optimum Times. Once you're aware of your Optimum Times and abilities you will find it easier to judge what you can achieve and when.

> **The plan is like having a daily life-coaching session!**

12. I am already doing a number of self-development techniques. Can I fit them into the plan?

Yes! This is exactly how I see women using the plan. The plan is a starting point, a model that you can shape to your own unique cycle and abilities. Use any self-development techniques when they are in tune with your Optimum Times, or adapt them to fit in with your natural abilities.

Where possible though, try to use techniques that help you to *accept* aspects of a particular phase that you may think of as bad or negative, rather than trying to *fix* them. It's not the phases of the cycle that are negative, but rather the way we approach them.

Chapter 9

The Optimized Woman Daily Plan

If you want to get ahead, get a cycle!

Plan outline

Dynamic phase

Cycle day 7: New energy!
Well-being action: Catching up on tasks.
Goal achievement action: Researching and groundwork.
Work enhancement action: Tackling complex issues and information.

Cycle day 8: Planning and analysis.
Well-being action: Getting healthy.
Goal action: Planning the month ahead.
Work enhancement action: Status analysis.

Cycle day 9: Starting projects.
Well-being action: Getting started.
Goal action: Pushing yourself.
Work enhancement action: Learning something new.

Cycle day 10: Individual empowerment.
Well-being action: Thought power.
Goal action: Creating feelings of success and fulfillment.
Work enhancement action: Focusing on yourself.

Cycle day 11: Positive belief.
Well-being action: Positive affirmations.
Goal action: Believing in the future.
Work enhancement action: Focusing on what you enjoy.

Cycle day 12: Righting wrongs.
Well-being action: Standing up.
Goal action: Imagining the knock-on effect.
Work enhancement action: Being a champion.

Cycle day 13: Setting up for the Expressive phase.
Well-being action: Reaching out.
Goal action: Nurturing your projects.
Work enhancement action: Feeling comfortable at work.

Expressive phase

Cycle day 14: Building success and confidence.
Well-being action: Positive day-dreaming.
Goal action: Creating the evidence.
Work enhancement action: Recognizing your successes.

Cycle day 15: Communication.
Well-being action: Accepting yourself.
Goal action: Seeking other viewpoints.
Work enhancement action: Evaluating people's needs.

Cycle day 16: Expressing appreciation.
Well-being action: Enjoying what you have.
Goal action: Appreciating the journey.
Work enhancement action: Appreciating others.

Cycle day 17: Compromise and balance.
Well-being action: Harmonizing your space.
Goal action: Creating win-win solutions.
Work enhancement action: Dealing with blocks and disputes.

Cycle day 18: Persuasion and networking.
Well-being action: Being actively sociable.
Goal achievement action: Contacting targeted support.
Work enhancement action: Networking.

Cycle day 19: Presenting ideas and selling concepts.
Well-being action: Gaining help and support.

Goal action: Selling your dream.

Work enhancement action: Selling your ideas.

Cycle day 20: Setting up for the Creative phase.

Well-being action: Organizing the week ahead.

Goal action: Identifying areas needing creativity.

Work enhancement action: Optimizing your resources.

Creative phase

Cycle day 21: Releasing your creativity.

Well-being action: Taking two-minute creative breaks.

Goal achievement action: Creating something physical.

Work enhancement action: Applying your creative flare.

Cycle day 22: Seeding the subconscious.

Well-being action: Mental 'Googling'!

Goal action: Looking for feedback and synchronicity.

Work action: Brainstorming.

Cycle day 23: Doing the small stuff.

Well-being action: Nurturing yourself.

Goal action: Taking small steps.

Work action: Doing the small stuff.

Cycle day 24: Preparing for the Reflective phase.

Well-being action: Creating free time.

Goal action: Prioritizing.

Work action: Creating scheduling solutions.

Cycle day 25: Slowing down.

Well-being action: Allowing your body to slow down.

Goal action: Being realistic.

Work enhancement action: Allocating more time.

Cycle day 26: Clearing the decks.
Well-being action: Clearing emotionally.
Goal action: Focusing your energy.
Work enhancement action: Clearing out.

Cycle day 27: Listening to our inner needs.
Well-being action: Listening to your needs.
Goal action: Focusing on underlying needs.
Work action: Taking nothing personally.

Reflective phase

Cycle day 28/1: Meditation and being.
Well-being action: Meditation.
Goal action: Letting go.
Work enhancement action: Working with your energies.

Cycle day 2: Touching base with our authentic self.
Well-being action: Dropping the baggage.
Goal action: Rediscovering fulfillment.
Work enhancement action: Being true to yourself.

Cycle day 3: Discovering the real priorities.
Well-being action: Changing 'shoulds' into 'coulds'.
Goal action: Refining your internal list.
Work action: Identifying pressure sources.

Cycle day 4: Letting go of resistance.
Well-being action: Accepting your inner connection.
Goal action: Discovering your resistance.
Work action: Taking a new direction.

Cycle day 5: Reviewing.
Well-being action: Reflecting on personal issues.

Goal action: Checking your progress.

Work enhancement action: Getting an overview.

Cycle day 6: Setting up for the Dynamic phase.

Well-being action: Choosing adventures.

Goal action: Targeting action.

Work action: Focusing your energies.

Dynamic phase

Day 7

Optimum Time for: New Energy!

Welcome to the *Dynamic* phase, the start of a new month. This month is going to be incredibly exciting as we journey through the different Optimum Times and use their associated abilities to help make the changes we need in order to create the success and fulfillment we desire. Every month we have the opportunity to build on what we have experienced and achieved in the previous month and to start afresh, leaving behind any emotional baggage, actions and expectations which haven't worked out the way we'd hoped.

Our month starts with a natural increase in our energies, enthusiasm and self-confidence. We have left our hibernation stage, and in the following days will feel the urge to get things done, catch up on tasks left unfinished in the *Reflective* phase, start new projects, stand up for what feels right, and to follow our heart.

We are able to bring the deep understanding and commitments we make in the *Reflective* phase out into the everyday world in the form of positive dynamic action.

The *Dynamic* phase is similar to the spring; it's a time to feed and water the seeds of new ideas, helping them to grow into the first green shoots. Later, in the *Expressive* phase, we can nurture the growth and pick the fruit; in the *Creative* phase, cut back the dead wood; and then in the *Reflective* phase acknowledge which new seeds to plant and grow again.

Well-being action: Catching up on Tasks

Enjoy your new source of dynamic energy and use this time to get things done. Look at the list of 'must dos' you created on day 3, or if you're just starting the plan make a list of the things which weren't completed last month and the tasks you want completed this month. How many could you accomplish this week? Remember, if a task is more appropriate to another phase, and timescales allow, make a diary note of when you plan to do it.

Also make a start on tasks that you have been meaning to do for months or even years. With your high energy levels you'll be able to make good progress in a short time and you'll lose the associated stress and guilt you've been carrying around.

Goal Achievement action: Researching and Groundwork

As well as experiencing increasing physical energy, your mental processes will also be getting sharper and quicker, so start to exercise your mind as well.

This is the Optimum Time to work out what actions you are going to take this month to achieve your goals. Research your approach by reading life-coaching books, books on success and fulfillment, and by searching and collating relevant information.

Try out goal achievement methods such as Neuro-Linguistic Programming (NLP), notice the techniques of the successful people around you, and consider how you could do the same.

Work Enhancement action: Tackling Complex Issues and Information

The *Dynamic* phase drive and its focus on goals and achievements can create a loss of empathy for other people. Actions and words can come across as being too focused, or even as aggressive and dictatorial. This is however a great time for practical analysis and planning – but it needs to be done alone before presenting the ideas to others. Making some space between your 'Eureka' moment and sharing your ideas allows your thoughts to slow to a more patient state in which to explain your solutions and plans.

Put aside some time alone today to work on any problems

which involve complex details, multiple aspects, timing, planning, structure and organization.

Dynamic phase

Day 8

Optimum Time for: Planning and Analysis

The *Dynamic* phase offers us the opportunity to take an overview perspective at the same time as focusing in on the little details. This makes it the Optimum Time to examine existing short term and long term plans, and to create new ones.

Life-coaching techniques ask us to think about our needs and goals in life and to determine where we're willing to put in the extra time and effort to achieve them. The previous phases will have given us a good idea about what's important to us and in which directions we should place our efforts.

Having chosen to commit to a main over-riding goal in the *Reflective* phase, we can focus the powers of our *Dynamic* phase mind on working through the stages we need to take in order to reach it. This is our long term action plan. We can then sub-divide each action into a number of tasks, starting with what we're going to do today.

Goals and action plans need a timescale in order to motivate us to make them happen. We can use this phase to think about when we would like to achieve our goal, and analyze whether it is realistic considering the list of actions and tasks required. The strong analytical and reasoning functions of this phase enable us to create lists of things to do without becoming emotionally overwhelmed, which can happen in the *Creative* phase. We have the opportunity to take an overview and break our goals down into exciting monthly, weekly, and daily tasks to keep us on track throughout the month.

Well-being action: Getting Healthy

In the *Creative* and *Reflective* phases you may have lost interest in going out, physical activity and living a healthy lifestyle. The enthusiasm and motivation of the *Dynamic* phase means that this is the Optimum Time to restart your diet, to set your weight or healthy eating targets for the month, and to plan your meals for the weeks ahead. Only ever weigh yourself once a month, and do it in this phase. Whatever the reading, you will have the positive self-image and the motivation to take it onboard.

Use your optimized planning skills to work out how you can get more exercise every day, fit in sessions in the gym or attend new classes such as yoga, Pilates or even belly-dancing! Planning and organizing now will help keep you motivated during your less energetic phases.

Your mind will also be ready to learn something new and eager to apply it, which makes this phase the best time to read self-development books and attend workshops and classes.

Goal action: Planning the Month Ahead

If you are just starting the plan, use your sharp mental abilities today to decide on a goal for this month and to create an action plan – a list of all the tasks you'll need to do to achieve it.

If you have already followed the Optimized Woman Daily Plan for a month, you will have reviewed the emotional commitment to your goals in the *Reflective* phase and can now use this Optimum Time to start planning your practical approach and timing for this month. You can factor in any changes in your goals over the last month, things which didn't get done from last month's action plan, and any changes in the timescales.

Use your diary, the Daily Plan, and your list of tasks to work out, where possible, the Optimum Times for doing each task. Obviously you can't always fit everything into your Optimum Times, but this doesn't mean that you can't complete your action plan; you'll just not be working precisely in tune with your enhanced abilities.

Work Enhancement action: Status Analysis

The *Dynamic* phase enhances your analytical abilities, which makes it an ideal time to examine the state of current projects and update schedules, milestones and deadlines. Analyze work activities such as filing and reporting, and design more efficient and effective methods of working.

Your enhanced mental abilities also mean you have the ability to focus on details, so use this time to check through the small print in contracts, formulate financial proposals, read through complex documents and write or edit reports.

Dynamic phase

Day 9

Optimum Time for: Starting Projects

When we start new projects unaware of our Optimum Times, we can be surprised and frustrated when we constantly seem to fail at achieving the desired outcome. For example, if we try to start a diet or to stop smoking in our *Creative* or *Reflective* phases, our low levels of energy, confidence and motivation mean that we are less likely to succeed. The more often we start a project at the wrong time and don't achieve our goal, the more likely our self-confidence and self-esteem will suffer. Obviously, the best time to start a project is when we have strong self-confidence and the energy to organize our lives to support the new project – the *Dynamic* phase.

The *Dynamic* phase offers us all the heightened abilities we need to get things started: high motivation, confidence in our ability, sharp mental skills and physical stamina. So often I hear women wishing they could remain in this phase throughout the whole month, but although the *Dynamic* phase is good for starting things it lacks the continuing supportive skills of the *Expressive* phase, the inspiration of the *Creative* phase, and the wisdom of the *Reflective* phase. When we make the most of our heightened abilities in their Optimum Times we are much more likely to achieve our goals and reach beyond our expectations.

Well-being action: Getting Started

This is the Optimum Time to start up new projects. Let your enthusiasm and drive today motivate you towards taking the first steps. A journey of a thousand miles starts with one step, so take action now.

Look at any current on-going projects and use your *Dynamic* phase to re-energize them or to start the next level or stage. If you're cutting down on smoking you could go to the next lower level of cigarettes, or if you're working out in the gym you could start increasing your times or repetitions. Don't miss out on this wonderful opportunity to **revitalize existing projects** and **start new ones**.

Goal action: Pushing yourself

You have done your planning (day 8). You have your list of tasks; now take action. In this phase, push yourself - your multi-tasking abilities and physical energy will be there to support you. You may find that your focus and driven energy can make people around you feel a little neglected or isolated. Take time to explain that this is your optimum week for action and you are simply making the best use of it to catch up on tasks or to get projects rolling. You will become more people-orientated when you enter into your *Expressive* phase.

Work Enhancement action: Learning Something New

The *Dynamic* phase can enhance your ability to learn things, so this is an ideal time to look at the manual you've been saying you should read, go on a work skills related course, or simply to ask someone to show you how to do something. When you are planning your month ahead, try to allocate some learning time into this phase. The *Dynamic* phase is not a particularly good phase for teamwork, so choose one-on-one courses, lectures, or book and computer learning. Try choosing subjects that you would normally think are too complex for you to learn; you may surprise yourself with how quickly you can pick things up in this phase.

Dynamic phase

Day 10

Optimum Time for: Individual Empowerment

The focus of this phase is very much on us as individuals. Very often with the pressures of work, responsibilities, people's opinions and our own inner criticisms we can lose touch with our sense of individuality, independence, and self-worth.

The *Dynamic* phase is the ideal time to activate our personal power, to feel that we have worth and to know we have the willpower to make things happen. This phase gives us permission to re-empower ourselves by validating our needs and dreams, to take the time and energy to express them, and most importantly to take actions towards fulfilling them. We are given permission to be self-centered and to put our needs foremost in our minds for consideration. Often when we acknowledge that our needs are important and commit the time to fulfilling them in this phase, we can experience a less disruptive *Creative* phase.

The *Dynamic* phase has a huge amount of vital energy which we can put behind our needs to manifest the outcomes. We can use our positive thoughts and attitude to attract the abundance, relationships, health, success and fulfillment we desire. Many of us have been brought up believing that to be 'good' we always have to put other people's needs ahead of our own, and because of this we can lose this unique opportunity once a month to recharge our self-worth and self-esteem batteries. It's the renewal of our personal power in this phase that can give us the required strength and self-belief to help others throughout the rest of the month.

Well-being action: Thought Power

You can actively harness the natural positive thought power experienced during this phase to create the things you want. To create more of something, simply focus your thoughts on what you already have, creating positive feelings of happiness and gratitude. These feelings in turn will attract more of what you want. Practice focusing on the glass being half full! A fun method of attracting abundance, from the book *The Secret* by Rhonda Byrne, is to write out a bank account paying-in slip with the amount that you wish to receive. Make the amount more than something you can imagine coming to you through normal means. Look at the slip every day, carry it with you, know that you have that money in your life and enjoy imagining spending it on all the things you desire. Feel happy, empowered, and grateful – this money is for you because you are worth it.

Goal action: Creating Feelings of Success and Fulfillment

When you increase your feelings of empowerment and success, you increase the belief that you will achieve your future goals.

The *Dynamic* phase is the Optimum Time for using a Neuro-Linguistic Programming (NLP) technique called 'anchoring'. This involves reliving or imagining a situation which creates positive feelings, and uses a physical trigger such as clapping or clicking your fingers to 'anchor' them. At a later date, such as in the *Creative* or *Reflective* phases when you may need to reconnect to more positive thoughts and beliefs, you can use your trigger to reconnect and experience more optimistic feelings.

Choose a memory, or imagine an outrageous situation, to create feelings of being happy, successful and confident. Make the experience as real as you can. Make the colors bright, the feelings intense and the sounds strong. When you've created a powerful experience, carry out your physical trigger, and then think of something boring and everyday. Now repeat the above process two more times to anchor the feelings to the physical trigger.

By setting up our anchoring in this Optimum Time we can boost its effectiveness and create stronger results in other phases.

Work Enhancement action: Focusing on Yourself

So often in the working environment it is necessary to work as part of a team. But a team only works well when the individual feelings and needs of the members are validated and met, and this includes you.

Focus on yourself today. Ask yourself what you need to do to enhance your work and your feelings of well-being at work. What can you do to meet your work needs? Who could you approach at work to help you?

If you need to approach other people to help you or to do something for you, wait until around day 19. In the *Expressive* phase we are much more able to express ourselves in non-critical and non-judgmental terms, and are more able to accept and understand people's responses.

Dynamic phase

Day 11

Optimum Time for: Positive Belief

During the *Dynamic* phase we are more receptive to believing positive thoughts about ourselves, the future or a particular situation. Unlike in the *Creative* phase, where using a positive affirmation can call forth numerous reasons for the statement used not being true, the *Dynamic* phase intrinsically provides deep feelings of belief in the statement. This makes the *Dynamic* phase the Optimum Time to use positive thought exercises to enhance our belief in our abilities, to validate ourselves and our dreams, and to build our confidence. Exercising this ability to believe once a month helps us to create deep impactful changes within ourselves and can help us to feel stronger when meeting the emotional or mental challenges later in the *Creative* and *Reflective* phases. We can also use the *Dynamic* phase to motivate ourselves by focusing on the outcomes of our goals. As we are naturally more able to believe in the positive, visualizing ourselves as succeeding becomes a very powerful tool to create the positive emotions needed to generate action, meet challenges, and keep the momentum going through those phases where we experience a less dynamic energy.

Well-being action: Positive Affirmations

The *Dynamic* phase is the Optimum Time to use positive affirmations for self-improvement and for manifesting desires. Positive affirmations are constructive statements about desired outcomes in language which suggests they exist already. For example, 'I am growing in happiness and fulfillment'. 'I am in the process of achieving all my goals with ease'. 'I am in the process of increasing my abundance'. 'I am growing in success'. 'My life is increasingly full of exciting opportunities'. 'I am growing in confidence every day'.

Decide on one affirmation for this month and write it down on a number of pieces of paper. Place your statement in locations where you will easily notice them. Take a few minutes each day to repeat your statement out loud, and really feel the emotions behind the words. When you have completed your affirmation, spend a moment feeling gratitude for your desires being fulfilled. Don't miss out on this monthly opportunity to recharge your self-empowerment batteries.

You can also use this practice to good effect in the *Expressive* phase.

Goal action: Believing in the Future

Take a few minutes today to visualize yourself with your goal completed.

What does it feel like? What are you doing differently to your current life? Who is in your life? Imagine the course of a day once your goal is completed. How do you feel when you get up? What is your routine? What do you do during the day? Who do you meet and where do you go? How do you feel when you go to bed at night?

Make your imagination as bright and as vibrant as possible, like the memory of a good day you have already experienced. Bask in these wonderful feelings.

Feel good about yourself and your goal, and take your internal images and positive feelings out into the everyday world to make it happen!

Work Enhancement action: Focusing on what you Enjoy

The working day often becomes so dominated by mundane tasks that it's difficult not to lose the initial enthusiasm, self-belief and vibrant energy experienced when you first started the job or the day. The *Dynamic* phase offers the opportunity to rekindle this enthusiasm by creating feelings of self-belief and by enhancing the positive feelings you have for the aspects of your work that you truly enjoy.

Look at your work; focus on what you enjoy and what brings fulfillment. Think about the skills and tasks you are good at and the knowledge you have, and experience the wonderful feelings of self-belief and confidence this brings. For today, believe in yourself and your work. Enjoy these positive feelings.

> # Dynamic phase
>
> ## Day 12

Optimum Time for: Righting Wrongs

The *Dynamic* phase brings with it a strong sense of 'right' and 'wrong'. In the *Expressive* and *Reflective* phases we are less likely to make a stand, but suddenly in the *Dynamic* phase it becomes important to fight for what we feel is right, and not just for ourselves but also for the injustices we see around us and in the world in general. We can feel much more assertive and more willing to take action on fairness, and on other people's behalf. It's the phase of the campaigner, the voice of fair play, the eco-warrior, the letter writing / telephoning complainant, and the defender of the victim.

When directed thoughtfully, our ability to take action based on our feelings can become the catalyst for major change. By taking a moral stance and taking a step towards acting on our principles we can feel that we are expressing our deepest beliefs and having a positive effect. It also provides positive feedback that we can make a difference in the world, and that we are empowered.

However, when not directed thoughtfully this phase can be one of dominating and aggressive behavior. Our feelings of injustice and conviction on what must be done to put things right can ride rough-shod over other people's feelings. So be careful.

Well-being action: Standing up

Think about what feels right or wrong in your everyday life. Where can you be more assertive about who you are, your ideas, your boundaries and what feels 'right' to you? Use your analytical and constructive mental abilities to work out how you can fix things and make situations feel right. Ask yourself if you have been fair or unfair towards others in the past month. Were your actions beneficial for both you and them? Don't just stand up for yourself; who around you needs help to fight their cause? Consider how you could make a difference. Remember this phase is good for initiating a project, structuring and planning a campaign, writing to people, creating a petition, and focusing on the details. Face-to-face meetings and supporting people in their own assertiveness is better suited to the *Expressive* phase.

Goal action: Imagining the knock-on Effect

One way to help you increase your personal motivation is to consider how achieving your goal is 'right' not just for yourself but also for others. Very often you can sabotage your goals by subconsciously feeling you are being 'selfish'. However, if you recognize that your happiness, well-being, financial security, fitness or success will benefit other people, you can feel truly worthy of achieving your goal.

Ask yourself if there is an altruistic aspect to achieving your goal? When you have achieved it, how will it have a positive effect on those around you? What would achieving your goal allow you to do that would benefit others? Make a quick note of all the benefits you can imagine and add to the list during the day as insights occur.

Work Enhancement action: Being a Champion

What feels 'right' and 'wrong' about your work? Are your co-workers treated fairly and with respect? Do the lines of communication work well? Is there enough support for colleagues, clients or customers? Is the company/employer/organization you are working for playing fair? Is it aligned with your ethical values?

What action can you take to fix problems or to make others aware of any problems? If you choose to take action, try to do it with the agreement of others. A hero rushing in to 'save the day' can be interpreted as being critical, dominating or aggressive.

Dynamic phase

Day 13

Optimum Time for: Setting up for the Expressive phase

As we journey from the *Dynamic* phase into the *Expressive* phase we become less focused on ourselves, less analytical, and less driven. We become more aware of other people's needs and the importance of connecting with others. We also become more empathic, more tolerant and more able to observe and understand feelings. Whereas in the *Dynamic* phase we are running with new ideas and projects, the *Expressive* phase gives us the opportunity to become more supportive and nurturing of the projects we have started. It is therefore the Optimum Time to help things to grow, and we have an intuitive knowledge of how to do it.

In this phase we can also be more tolerant, giving us the ability to really listen to what people say and to give empathic responses, making this the Optimum Time for us to support friends, family members and work colleagues. When people feel that their feelings and needs have been heard and validated they are more willing to create positive relationships, whether it's within a family or within a team meeting. Our own positive feelings of confidence and strength, plus our communication skills in this phase, make this the Optimum Time to nurture relationships.

This phase sees a change in our creativity from the mental activity of the *Dynamic* phase to a more practical, hands-on, emotional, 'motherly' creativity. Don't waste this exciting Optimum Time; use it to create the care you need and the supportive environment you want, and to creatively express the person you feel you are.

Well-being action: Reaching out

Make a list of people you haven't contacted for a while or given enough time to recently. During the *Expressive* phase you have enough emotional strength and stability to support more people than you think. Commit to 'reaching out and touching' someone in the next week. Who around you needs extra care and attention? Perhaps you've been neglecting them during your *Dynamic* phase. How can you help them feel more nurtured and supported during the next week?

Goal action: Nurturing your Projects

Look at any projects and goals which at the moment seem to be stuck, going off course, or which are losing momentum. Think about what you could do to support them, to create new positive momentum, or to help them to develop. Do they need a bit of your attention on a regular basis? Do you need to commit more time and effort to supporting them than you're doing at the moment? Projects and goals tend to fade and die unless you continually nurture them with your energies, actions and attention.

Work Enhancement action: Feeling Comfortable at Work

The workplace is the place you spend a large proportion of your day. How you feel about your working environment affects how you feel about your work and how well you work. Look round the space where you spend most of your time. Is there anything you could do to make it feel more supportive, comfortable or homely? Something as simple as a plant can help.

If you are working in an area that you cannot change, or you are always on the move, what can you do with your clothes / bag / briefcase to support and express your femininity? Have fun planning your clothes for the week ahead or the changes you're going to make to your working environment.

End of Dynamic phase summary

To help you assess your experiences during your *Dynamic* phase, you may like to answer the following questions.

1. How did you experience your *Dynamic* phase? In comparison to the *Reflective* phase, how did you feel?

Emotionally	
Mentally	
Physically	

2. On which days of the plan did you feel that the information and actions were in-tune with your personal experiences?

3. Which abilities did you find enhanced or easier in this phase compared to the previous one?

4. How did you practically apply your heightened abilities this month?

5. What are you planning to do with these Optimum Time abilities next month?

6. What was the most surprising, intriguing or amazing thing you discovered about yourself in this phase?

Personalizing the plan

You can personalize the Optimized Woman Daily Plan to suit

your own unique cycle by choosing actions from the plan which were in-tune with your Optimum Time abilities and listing them against your cycle date. You can repeat individual actions over a number of days.

Fill in the table below and see if you can plan some tasks for next month which will make the best use of your enhanced abilities.

Dynamic Phase		
My Optimum Time for:		
Cycle day number	Optimum Time actions	Planned task for next month

Expressive phase

Day 14

Optimum Time for: Building Success and Confidence

Welcome to the *Expressive* phase, your opportunity to build feelings of success, to create supportive relationships and to express your ideas and dreams to the world.

We often have so many responsibilities and tasks that we never seem to reach the end of the 'to do' list. The only success we tend to allow ourselves is the satisfaction that we have cleared X% off the list before we fall asleep exhausted. We lose out on the reality of success in our lives, missing out on the feelings of a job well done. We also frequently define success only in terms of life-shattering events, so it's not surprising that we feel unhappy, disempowered, and lacking the sense of motivation generated by feelings of personal achievement.

When we do take time to think about the things that we have achieved, we not only feel good about ourselves but we also see ourselves as actively empowered and expressing who we are in the world. Our successes can be small or large, important only to us or seen as having a positive effect on friends, family or the whole world! By building a baseline of success feelings each month, we start to create the evidence that we are successful, and we begin to experience more self-confidence and higher self-esteem.

The *Expressive* phase is very feelings-orientated, so it is easier for us in this phase than in any other phase to generate positive feelings of success.

Our subconscious self cannot determine the difference between the real and imagined, so we can feel imagined successes as real. We can also rewrite past failures into past achievements!

For example, if an important event a few years ago didn't go well, rewrite the past and instead experience positive emotions of success. We will still have learned from the original experience, but why not carry a more positive, empowering story of the past rather than a negative one? By doing this we can build a strong foundation of success feelings which will powerhouse our motivation.

Well-being action: Positive Day-dreaming

Make up a totally imaginary event in which you are successful, or rewrite a past experience in your mind. It can be as fanciful as you like, so have fun. Imagine the event as vividly as you can; make the colors bright, feel textures, and hear the sounds. This is an event happening to you right now, and your mind will take the memory of it and its accompanying feelings into your future. Allow yourself to really enjoy the exquisite pleasures of success, achievement and well-being. Put the power of positive day-dreaming into your life.

Goal action: Creating the Evidence

Positive affirmations can be used effectively during the *Expressive* phase and by adding the term 'because' at the end of the statement, they become even more powerful. For example you could add a previous success as emotional evidence to the affirmation 'I feel successful because ...'

You can also make your affirmations more powerful and emotive by adding the term 'I love'. For example: 'I love having money in my life'. Your subconscious is more receptive in this phase to positive emotions as actual evidence for something being real. By adding positive emotions to your affirmations, you help fix the new concepts in both your emotional patterns and your mental processes.

Today use your Optimum Time for feelings to help you to generate a strong belief in your ability to be successful. Do this by creating evidence of your successes:

'I feel successful because ... (*add your evidence*). I love being successful'.

When you feel successful you will have more motivation and inner strength to see your goal through the challenges ahead.

Work Enhancement action: Recognizing your Successes

Use today to answer the question 'What have I achieved at work and how have I helped and supported my company / co-workers / clients / customers?'

Focus on the small everyday things you have achieved as well as any bigger accomplishments. Doing small things for other people very often slips through our success recognition net, and even doing things you had to do, or didn't want to do, still count as successes.

This process can turn a seemingly dull job without achievement into one full of accomplishment. By proving to yourself that you are successful, you immediately enhance and support your motivation and enthusiasm.

Expressive phase

Day 15

Optimum Time for: Communication

The *Expressive* phase is the Optimum Time to find out how other people are thinking and feeling. The caring and selfless tendencies of this nurturing phase mean that we are less likely to feel overly sensitive to other people's attitudes or threatened by their opinions, words and needs. This phase includes a natural ability to communicate well, to accept people for who they are, to validate their priorities and opinions, and to be an empathic and active listener. We can use our enhanced aptitude to listen in order to find out what other people feel about their lives. With so little spare time in our busy schedules we very rarely put aside the time needed to really listen to what our children, our partner, family, friends, co-workers, clients or customers say to us.

Simply just stopping what we are doing, turning towards another person and giving them our full attention can be enough to create a more positive relationship. Add to this giving them the time and freedom to talk, and we can be surprised at the assumptions we've been making about how they feel and what they need.

We can also ask people what they need in order to have a better relationship with us, and how we can help to enrich their lives, without having to defend past actions or perceived attacks on ourselves. Unlike the *Creative* phase, where we are more likely to take things personally, and the *Dynamic* phase where we're more action-orientated and less empathic, communication in the *Expressive* phase is easier, more positive and with less need for us to get our view across.

Well-being action: Accepting Yourself

To support others you also need to support yourself, and the positive 'motherly' feelings of the *Expressive* phase can be used to encourage self-acceptance and positive thoughts. For many women, their internal dialogue often consists of self-criticism and the identification of their faults and mistakes, but the 'inner mother' aspect of the *Expressive* phase can offer the wonderful opportunity to reconnect to feelings of unconditional self acceptance and love.

Today, use the following affirmation to give yourself permission to be whatever and whoever you are: 'I let myself be ...' You could add 'beautiful', 'successful', 'happy', 'loved' or any other aspect of yourself that needs feelings of validation, nurturing and acceptance. You may like to continue using this affirmation throughout the phase.

Goal action: Seeking other Viewpoints

The *Expressive* phase is the Optimum Time for asking other people for their views and perspectives on your goals and progress, as at this time you can take on board their comments without interpreting them as criticism. Find someone to give an outside viewpoint on what you are trying to achieve. This could simply be a close friend for a personal overview, or it could be an expert with particular experience and knowledge about your goal. Be specific about the type of feedback that you'd like from them. In particular, concentrate on areas where you feel stuck or unsure, as very often your reaction to what someone says can clarify how you truly feel about a situation.

Work Enhancement action: Evaluating People's Needs

This is a great time to review working relationships and take part in job and staff evaluations. Ask co-workers or employees about their work, and if there's anything they would like changed to create a better working environment and a sense of appreciation.

Get personal, and find out what co-workers and bosses need from you. Yes, it's likely to come across as sounding critical of you, but remember that during this phase you are more able to see their point of view and are less likely to take anything said as a personal attack on your or your work. You are also more able to hear the need behind the words and the feelings they are expressing.

Expressive phase

Day 16

Optimum Time for: Expressing Appreciation

Throughout the *Expressive* phase our sense of personal well-being can be connected to expressing our feelings of love and appreciation, gratitude and caring.

The well-being of our relationships with people we know, with strangers, with communities and with the planet, can become important to us. Unlike in the *Creative* phase where we can easily become overwhelmed by other people's lives and needs, in this phase our natural empathy and inner strength empowers us to take supportive action.

One way of taking supportive action is to express appreciation and gratitude.

Appreciation of the plight of the planet makes us put the bottles in the recycling bank. Appreciation of our co-workers leads to building better relationships and creates motivation. Expressing gratitude for help and support, or simply because a person is part of our lives, helps others to feel important and valued and creates long-lasting relationships.

Unlike the *Dynamic* phase, which drives us to new directions and projects, the *Expressive* phase lends itself to appreciating our lives as they are now. We can experience a greater appreciation for the work we do, the environment we live in, and the relationships we have. The *Expressive* phase also gives us the patience to watch our current projects grow and develop in their own way, and the ability to create change through gentle nurturing and guidance rather than through dramatic change.

Well-being action: Enjoying what you Have

Concentrate on simply enjoying the life you have. Feel happy and grateful for all the rich experiences you're having, for the people, places and objects you love, and for everything which enriches your life.

Look around at nature and appreciate the senses you have to enjoy the world, and simply enjoy being alive. Ask yourself 'What do I love in my life, about my life and about myself?' Enjoy what you love and you will attract more.

Goal action: Appreciating the Journey

Achieving your goals can sometimes make you so focused on the happy event in the future that you forget to live the journey. You forget to stop and look around at where you have come from, how far you have traveled, and how beautiful the path is you are walking. Appreciating your journey and how it enriches you can fill you with the motivation to keep going when you face challenges.

Forget about taking action towards achieving your goals; allow them the space to develop in their own time and in their own way. By giving them this freedom you may be surprised at the outcome. Also forget about future successes; today simply feel gratitude for where you stand on your path.

Work Enhancement action: Appreciating Others

Who at work has been doing a good job? Who has helped you in your own work?

If you are involved in a team or a group, identify which members are not being appreciated enough for their input. Who around you stands out as not appreciating the effort, skills, and commitment they themselves have put in?

Think up ways you can express your appreciation. These could be anything from a simple thank you card to creating a monthly team award.

Expressive phase

Day 17

Optimum Time for: Compromise and Balance

The *Expressive* phase can offer us gifts of heightened empathy, an awareness of connections and relationships, and an insightful perception of people's needs.

These skills and abilities make this the Optimum Time to arbitrate in disputes, and create win-win situations, compromises and balance. We are natural mediators, having the impartiality to understand the underlying factors influencing people's actions, feelings and the language they use.

Blocks in communication can often occur where people are unable to articulate their issues effectively; our Expressive phase abilities mean that we can help them to express themselves fully. Often this can facilitate 'outside the box' solutions, dispute break-throughs, changes in people's attitudes and new creative ideas.

It is also easy during this phase to tune into our inherent sense of harmony, but very often we don't take this awareness any further. The *Expressive* phase gives us the ability not only to feel what is out of harmony but also to feel what actions are needed to restore it within our environment and relationships.

Well-being action: Harmonizing your Space

Look around the room and tune into your sense of balance and harmony by asking yourself what feels uncomfortable about the space.

Does this space feel harmonious? Does it express yourself, and the other people who may share it in a way which is balanced? Choose one small thing which needs changing to bring harmony. How can you change it? Now go do it!

Goal action: Creating Win-Win Solutions

When working towards your goals situations arise where your desired outcome depends on other people's decisions and actions. When your rate of progress seems to be blocked by these people it can lead to uncomfortable feelings of powerlessness. Create win-win situations to get the results you want by adapting solutions to the needs you perceive beneath people's objections and obstruction.

The *Expressive* phase gives you the abilities you require to understand people's attitudes and needs in order to create win-win solutions which will motivate the other person to take the action you desire. At the moment, who is blocking or delaying your expected progress towards your goals? What could be the reason behind their action or inaction? Think of a win-win situation, and suggest it to the person involved. Ask them what they need, but be prepared to be flexible or to change your expectations.

Work Enhancement action: Dealing with Blocks and Disputes

This is the Optimum Time to deal with disputes, deadlocks and negotiations. It could be that you're having problems with a fellow worker, or progress on a project has broken down, or that you're involved in contractual negotiations.

Act as an external mediator in disputes and misunderstandings. If you are personally involved in a dispute, check your priorities. Compromise will mean letting go of or changing some of your needs.

Use your current abilities to recognize disharmony in teams and work situations, and to present possible solutions to those involved.

Expressive phase

Day 18

Optimum Time for: Persuasion and Networking

Have you ever wondered when would be the best time to ask for a raise or something you really want? That time is now! As well as emotional confidence and good communication skills, the *Expressive* phase also offers us the awareness and patience to get what we want through gentle persuasion.

Unlike the direct and impatient approach of the *Dynamic* phase, when we are more likely to offer a 'take it or leave it' ultimatum, the *Expressive* phase approach can consist of a subtle strategy to bring someone round to our point of view. We can use our increased awareness and empathy to tailor our approach to the person we want to persuade, or to plant an idea or run a targeted campaign to get what we want.

Our increased sociability during this phase also means that we can use casual situations to our advantage.

Networking can be daunting for many of us at any time, but the confidence of the *Expressive* phase means that we are more willing to take the first step. Talk to people; anyone and everyone. Contact clients, suppliers or work colleagues to help them to see our good points and how much we are supporting or helping them. Even if client or supplier management isn't our job, we can take extra time during this phase to contact them to thank them or to check that they're happy. We can also contact the departments or people who support us and say thank you for their input. It does sound like running a personality campaign, but as it evolves from the caring and nurturing abilities of the *Expressive* phase it's a genuine expression of who and what we are.

Well-being action: Being Actively Sociable

You can use this Optimum Time of sociability and networking by stepping outside of your usual environment and talking to the new people you meet as a consequence.

Try doing something you wouldn't normally do; change a routine, go to classes, or even throw a party. Make the commitment to introduce yourself to new people at any and every opportunity.

This is the time to support the people who support you, so go through your list of friends and family and commit to contacting at least one person you haven't heard from or seen recently. You could even invite them to the party.

Goal Achievement action: Contacting Targeted Support

Identify three people, organizations or businesses that could help you in your goal achievement. Think up a strategy for making first contact. Can you build your contact in stages? What form of contact would they most likely respond to? What would hook them in to being interested? What do you offer which would make them help you? How can you stand out? Take the first step towards contacting them today.

Work Enhancement action: Networking

Network by asking colleagues, clients and relevant businesses to introduce you to the people you need to know. Join industry groups or business clubs, go to conferences and events associated with your work, carry business cards to hand out to everyone you meet, and talk to strangers. Ask yourself if there is anything you need at work, and how could you get it by gentle persuasion. Can you plant an idea and make someone think that it's their own? Also think about how you can change the image people have of your work. Run your personal campaign throughout the *Expressive* phase!

Expressive phase

Day 19

Optimum Time for: Presenting Ideas and Selling Concepts

The emotional strength, confidence and communication abilities of the *Expressive* phase make it the Optimum Time to present our ideas and to sell anything from concepts to products, services and solutions. Not only do we have the ability to articulate and express a concept well, but because we are also more empathic about our audience's needs we are able to effectively adapt our delivery accordingly.

This means that we are more able to be constructive contributors in meetings, to teach and mentor, to deliver presentations and proposals, and to staff exhibition stands and the shop floor. Our enhanced receptiveness to our audience's needs means we can easily adapt to take in new parameters and viewpoints, making this an ideal time for customer service and sales and marketing.

It is also the Optimum Time to approach family members with new ideas about changes in routine, work/life balance, and your needs and expectations. Whatever we are selling, whether it's an idea which affects our family, a viewpoint in a meeting, or a product, we are actually selling ourselves at the same time. The *Expressive* phase enables us to justify our position, beliefs and activities without becoming aggressive or defensive in response, even in intensely negative environments. So if we have decided to leave our jobs, backpack round the world, start our own business or change something fundamental in our life, now is the time to mention it to anyone it may affect.

The *Expressive* phase is an Optimum Time for job interviews, writing our CV, and cold calling companies about potential work. Our natural optimism about ourselves and our abilities means we will come across well.

Well-being action: Gaining Support

We all have ideas on what others could do to help improve the quality of our lives. It could be giving more help and support, reducing their demands and expectations on us, being more understanding or doing more things which make us feel good.

Today take one idea and consider how you could present it to the people involved. Take into account their feelings and needs, and find a positive benefit they would get from your idea. Can you present the idea straight up, or do you need to take a subtle approach and build up to the idea? Don't worry about rejection; with your *Expressive* phase abilities you are patient and flexible enough to bring them round.

Note that you will need to take action today, before you start your *Creative* phase, or you could make this a project for your *Expressive* phase next month.

Goal action: Selling your Dream

All goals start with a dream. One way you can help your goal to manifest is to sell this dream and your ideas on how to achieve it to someone who can help. Start by defining your whole dream in a maximum of three sentences. This can be hard. Depending on how confident you feel, test it out on a family member, a friend or a work colleague. Every time you present your idea you not only develop a better understanding of what you have in mind but you're also more able to present it in a meaningful way. Use their questions to help you to refine your proposal for future presentations.

Work Enhancement action: Selling your Ideas

What ideas do you have about your work and working

environment? Can you see how to improve things or see opportunities and solutions missed by others? How well a new idea is received often depends on the working environment. Can you share your ideas in a meeting or in an informal phone call or email? What would help you to present your idea? Do you need diagrams, a mock-up, or quotes from other people?

Who really needs to know about your idea to (a) give you the recognition you deserve for it and (b) take action on it? With your natural *Expressive* phase charisma, no one is too high to reach.

Expressive phase

Day 20

Optimum Time for: Setting up for the Creative phase

The *Creative* phase is the 'big bad' time of the month for many women and it can be very obvious when it begins. For other women this phase develops more gradually, so it can be more difficult to identify when to start planning for the change in abilities. Like the *Dynamic* phase, the *Creative* phase is full of dynamic energy, only this time it is less logical and rational and more creative, emotional, explosive and intuitive.

This phase can announce its arrival with an increasing determination to get things done, an inability to let go or relax, and increasing levels of intolerance and frustration. We can also experience uncontrollable cascading thoughts, which can be negative or positively creative depending on our original seed thought.

As the *Creative* phase progresses our levels of mental focus and patience can drop, creating frustration and anger if we can't find things or have the information we need readily to hand. To help prevent this we can use the end of the *Expressive* phase to review the tasks and projects of the week ahead, and locate or create everything we are going to need in advance. This may involve asking other people to supply information to us early, or creating job-specific piles of items and documents. Keep in mind 'the five-minute rule':

> **Anything you can't find within 5 minutes will really bug you big time!**

While reviewing the week ahead we can compare the tasks with our Optimum Time abilities and see if we can reschedule anything to a better time for us. Remember; try to avoid conflict or sensitive situations, and to reduce your expectations of your levels of concentration and stamina the closer you get to the end of your phase. If you can't move meetings or deadlines, then set up some support systems, carry a notebook to write down ideas as they come to you, and be prepared to say to people 'I will get back to you on that' to give yourself more thinking space.

Identify creative projects to think about during the *Creative* phase. Don't lose out on this amazingly creative time to work on ideas and goals as well as blue-sky-thinking work projects and solutions. Finally, organize physical activities to release pent-up stress and frustrations as and when they peak.

Well-being action: Organizing the Week Ahead

Think about the week ahead and what needs doing. Try to use the days at the beginning of the phase to get as much out of the way as possible in the awareness that you may have less physical and mental energy to spare towards the end of the phase.

Also be aware that as the phase progresses you may experience physical changes in your stamina, need for sleep and nutritional requirements, as well as in your emotional needs. You many need to change your exercise regime to meet your energy highs and lows, alter your diet, go to bed earlier, and avoid particular people or sensitive subjects. Keep this in mind as you plan your life over the next week.

Goal action: Identifying areas Needing Creativity

The *Creative* phase is the Optimum Time for creative ideas and for cutting away the irrelevant or not useful. To keep the phase controlled and focused, identify areas within your goals where you need creative inspiration – it could be writing a business plan or an advert, working out a new approach or creating a new opportunity.

Also look for areas and approaches which have been unproductive, so you can use your optimum 'throwing out' time to change direction.

Work Enhancement action: Optimizing your Resources

Follow 'the five-minute rule' and assemble everything you will need to get jobs done over the next week. Look over your schedules and identify anything which could clash with your *Creative* phase abilities, such as group activities, negotiations, people management, and projects requiring logical and structured thought processes. If it's not possible to reschedule, think about how you can support yourself in these activities.

Also identify areas where you need creative thinking and ideas. This could include problem solving, presenting information in a different way, or simply running with an idea and seeing how you could make it work. Note down any projects which are not working well and may need major re-organizing. Finally, see if there are any places which need to be tidier and less cluttered.

By noting these points now you will have a list of positive and practical projects to act as a release for any frustrated energies if they arise.

End of Expressive phase summary

To help you assess your experiences during your *Expressive* phase, you may like to answer the following questions.

1. How did you experience your *Expressive* phase? In comparison to the *Dynamic* and *Reflective* phases, how did you feel?

Emotionally	
Mentally	
Physically	

2. On which days of the plan did you feel that the information and actions were in tune with your personal experiences?

3. Which abilities did you find enhanced or easier in this phase compared to the previous one?

4. How did you practically apply your heightened abilities this month?

5. What are you planning to do with the abilities of the *Expressive* phase next month?

6. What was the most surprising, intriguing or amazing thing you discovered about yourself in this phase?

Personalizing the plan

You can personalize the plan to suit your own cycle by choosing the actions which are in-tune with your Optimum Time abilities and listing them against your cycle date. You can repeat individual actions over a number of days.

Fill in the table below and see if you can plan some tasks for next month which will make the best use of your enhanced abilities.

Expressive Phase		
My Optimum Time for:		
Cycle day number	Optimum Time actions	Planned task for next month

Creative phase

Day 21

Optimum Time for: Releasing your Creativity

Welcome to the *Creative* phase, our opportunity to release our creative energies and ride an exciting wave of inspiration and intuition.

Unfortunately, many of us ignore our monthly surge of creativity, or misread the tension and frustration produced by our unfulfilled need to create as a sign of something wrong, either with ourselves or with our lives.

How many of us would describe ourselves as 'creative'? Not many, but only because we tend to have a limited definition of 'creativity'.

The menstrual cycle itself is a cycle of changing forms of creativity; we have the mental creativity of the *Dynamic* phase, the ability to create relationships and understanding in the *Expressive* phase, and the ability to create new life paths and new direction in the *Reflective* phase.

In the *Creative* phase we experience a more recognizable creativity – the ability and need to create something in the physical world, including creating a new 'look' for ourselves. When we completely change our wardrobe, or our hairstyle, the chances are it's in our *Creative* phase.

This phase is the Optimum Time to apply our creative energies to all areas of our lives and to enjoy the process. We can try out new activities just for the fun of it, and possibly discover new talents we never knew we had.

Although we can apply our creativity to many different projects, the *Creative* phase is not so much about the **product** but more about **being engaged** in an activity which lets our creative energies flow. It doesn't matter that the result of our creativity isn't perfect, or that it has no practical or commercial application, or that it ends up in the garbage. Once we start releasing our creativity we find that it responds by flowing freely, bringing feelings of calm, grounding and contentment not normally associated with the pre-menstrual phase.

Well-being action: Making two-minute Creative Breaks

It is possible to lessen feelings of frustration and tension in this phase by releasing your creative energies quickly and simply in small amounts during the day. Choose a creative activity for the next few days which you can easily do in two-minute breaks. You could doodle, color patterns, make up a song, write a poem or story, or do some needlework. In the busy, highly pressurized work environment it may seem strange for a female CEO to take some knitting out of a desk drawer for a two-minute creative break. Try it and see what happens to your feelings of well-being during this phase.

Goal Achievement action: Creating Something Physical

Identify areas where you can use your creativity to make something physical. You could draw a flowchart or a mindmap to show how your goals and tasks interconnect. If your goal involves a new business, try a quick sketch of a logo, or if it involves a product, play at designing the packaging or a leaflet. Write down any ideas; make them physical and not just thoughts. Find images of your goal and the things you want to achieve, and paste them on to a sheet of card – scissors and glue are creative tools.

Work Enhancement action: Applying your Creative Flair

This is the Optimum Time for working on any aspect of your job that needs creative input. Why not use this time for creating presentation visuals, mock-ups and new products, or for writing creative copy.

Apply your design skills to documents or marketing materials, to your Curriculum Vitae, your office decor or even your work clothes.

At this time creativity can be very intuitive, so trust your choices. You may not know at the time why something works, but later you may discover that your subconscious will provide you with the reasons.

Be aware that the creativity of this phase can get very focused, with a need for perfection, and letting go can be very difficult if you feel unhappy with the outcome of your work. When you find that you're not achieving good creative results quickly and easily, it's a sign that the Optimum Time for this type of creativity is passing.

Creative phase

Day 22

Optimum Time for: Seeding the Subconscious

So many of us experience thought avalanches during this phase, but we can take positive advantage of this creative ability by 'seeding the subconscious'.

These times of bombarding thoughts can feel overwhelming and out of our control, especially when the seed thought activating them is negative about our lives or about ourselves. If we step back and see this process as a wonderful creative capability which allows us to access the deep inner processing of our subconscious, we can use this ability practically to brainstorm ideas, solve problems and make 'Eureka' connections! We can control the direction of our subconscious creativity with questions and topics for new ideas, solutions and information.

We can think of the 'seeding' process as our conscious mind typing a question or a subject into our deeper 'computer' brain. We then get an hourglass symbol displayed on our mental screen as the request or subject is being processed.

After a while our computer brain will come back to us with insights, information, connections, ideas, solutions, images, words, impulses or inner knowing. We will have our 'wow!' moment.

Actively working with this ability is fun and wonderfully exciting. The ideas and thoughts can return from processing at any time and very rarely stay 'on screen' for very long, which means that we need to record the idea in some way when it occurs. A good habit is to carry around a small notebook in a pocket or a handbag. Very often the process of writing triggers more connections, more ideas and more inspiration.

> **The subconscious loves an interactive audience!**

Well-being action: Mental 'Googling'

Select a single problem you want to solve, and ask your computer brain for insight and solutions. Now find something fairly mindless to do, such as washing up, or go for a walk round the block. Concentrate on your action and allow your brain to process. Your subconscious will respond by sending you the odd thought about your problem. Run with the thoughts as they arise and see what happens.

At this early stage in the *Creative* phase, this process will be creative and positive. However, if you find that your 'seeding' starts a cascade of negative self-thought, leave this activity for its next Optimum Time - the *Reflective* phase.

Goal action: Looking for Feedback and Synchronicity

Pick a topic. Choose something for which you need inspiration or more information, or something which fills you with enthusiasm. It doesn't have to be specifically connected to your goals. Allow your subconscious to process the topic over the next few days and actively look out for any feedback or synchronicity from the world around you. Once your subconscious knows you are actively waiting for an answer, it will very happily interact with you! You may even find that it will make connections between unrelated topics and your goals. The ideas can come at any time and you can lose them quickly, so note them down even if you are sure you'll remember.

Work action: Brainstorming

What in your work needs a bit of brainstorming or 'out-of-the-box' thinking? Do you have any problems or areas which need an injection of new ideas, a new approach, or a different way of doing things? If nothing comes to mind, deliberately use this time to seed your consciousness with the question of how you can use this Optimum Time ability. Today, and over the next few days, give your computer mind some processing time dedicated to these problems or areas. Try staring blankly out of the window on the commuter train or when standing at the coffee making machine, or go for a short walk at lunchtime. You could even take the headphones off when you use the gym and use boredom to help you process.

Creative phase

Day 23

Optimum Time for: Doing the Small Stuff

The *Creative* phase brings together the active focus of the *Dynamic* phase with the emotions of the *Expressive* phase. But with reducing physical stamina and sometimes extreme emotional sensitivity, it can often feel like a time of little emotional control and of low self-esteem. We can easily lose touch with our feelings of being grounded, of success and fulfillment, of love and personal power.

The key to balancing this phase is to do small simple things to nurture ourselves and to stay grounded. We need to have activities which will help us detach from any negative self-thoughts, focus us inward as protection from times of extreme empathy, and create positive feelings of achievement and self-worth.

We can make a list in advance of things to do in this phase by looking around for small activities or by taking a larger task and splitting it down into simple steps. To generate feelings of being centered, successful and empowered, we need to choose small jobs that won't take long and don't involve a lot of input from other people (we can get frustrated in this phase if people don't do what we want when we want). In particular, anything that creates order can be particularly satisfying and create a sense of fulfillment and self-worth. By taking one simple task at a time and giving it all our attention we can lose ourselves in the activity, creating peaceful relief from any negative thoughts and protection from any outside emotional triggers. When we finish the task we have the added bonus of feelings of fulfillment and personal power.

The beauty of this phase is that we take our natural ability to 'mono-task' and withdraw, and positively use it to focus on and happily complete jobs which we would normally feel are monotonous and uninteresting.

Well-being action: Nurturing Yourself

Nurture your feelings of self-worth and fulfillment with small simple jobs which can be completed easily, like clearing out a drawer or kitchen cupboard, or by spending an evening relaxing in a bath with bubble bath, candles, soft music and chocolates!

What simple activities would make you feel nurtured and centered today? Do you need to switch off the news reports and soaps and avoid hearing about people's problems to protect your emotional sensitivity? Do you need some 'me' time or a little luxury in your life? What activity could you give your whole attention to, and feel self-worth as a result?

Goal action: Taking Small Steps

When we lose our sense of self-worth and success it can have a negative effect on our progress towards our goals. It is very important that we realize that any feelings of being overwhelmed or of inadequacy that we experience in this phase will pass. Any negative thoughts we have about our goals and our activities are simply thoughts, and our perception will change again as our phase changes. This is not the phase for making any major changes about our goals, so we need to keep our thoughts focused on the small details rather than the bigger picture. Take the list of tasks you have for your goal and split one item down into its smallest incremental steps. One step could be as simple as 'buy a stamp'. Focus on doing these small tasks one at a time, and ignore anything else. With each task completed, you will feel the success of a step forward. Remember that you will check in the *Reflective* phase to see if you're heading in the right direction, so don't worry about it for now.

Work action: Doing the Small Stuff

What small or boring tasks have you been putting off doing? Is there filing to be done, boxes to stack, an in-tray to sort through, a room to organize, or perhaps some photocopying or some other monotonous task to be done?

Don't write out a 'to do' list as this will generate pressure to get everything done and can enhance any feelings of being overwhelmed by tasks. However, once you've completed one small task. Look around and see if there's something else you can do, or refer back to the projects you outlined in Day 20.

Creative phase

Day 24

Optimum Time for: Preparing for the Reflective phase

The 'preparation for the next phase' day comes earlier in the *Creative* phase than in the others, as we're less likely to have the mental and physical energy to spare later in the week. As we enter the *Reflective* phase we can begin a time of letting go, of inner calm and of insight. It's a phase of the withdrawal of our emotional, mental and physical energies into hibernation, and of rejuvenation and restoration.

If we fight this new phase by expecting to carry on as 'normal', we fight our bodies and miss out on an Optimum Time for some powerfully transformative abilities.

The *Reflective* phase is our Optimum Time for reviewing how we feel about ourselves, about who we want to be and where we want to go in life. It's the time for making new commitments and starting new directions.

We can't reach the level of awareness the *Reflective* phase offers if we're running around meeting deadlines, responsibilities and expectations, so we need to delegate, let go of perfection and control, and to ask others to shoulder more for a few days.

To take advantage of this Optimum Time we need to make room in our lives to think, feel and simply 'be'. We can do this by looking ahead in our diaries at our tasks, responsibilities and schedules, and prioritizing activities to ensure that we have more relaxation time at least for cycle days one to four. It helps to remember that we will have more physical and mental energy in the *Dynamic* phase to catch up.

Well-being action: Creating Free Time

Ask others in advance to take over some of your normal activities, responsibilities and chores in cycle days one to four. By letting them know now, you're giving them plenty of time to adjust their own schedules and their expectations of what you will do. Also see if you can avoid social events, hectic schedules or demanding situations, so you can factor in more time alone to nurture yourself.

Goal action: Prioritizing

The *Reflective* phase is very important for helping us review our goals and our progress towards them. Not allocating quiet time for reflection during this phase means that we miss out on an extremely powerful opportunity to know what's right for us and to either commit to a new direction or to reaffirm the one we have already taken. Look through your schedules and tasks, and prioritize. Knowing that you will experience a reduction in mental and physical energy over the next week gives you the opportunity to put the energy you do have now into your top priority actions. By being ahead of schedule you can allow yourself the relaxation time you need to review during the *Reflective* phase.

Work action: Creating Scheduling Solutions

The last few days of the *Creative* phase and the first few days of the *Reflective* phase can be a real struggle when you have deadlines piling up and little mental and physical energy to deal with them.

If you force yourself to keep going during this time, you will lose the insightful opportunity that this phase brings. Use today to go through your schedules for the next eight days. Where possible, make your first two menstruation days as free from pressure and physical demands as you can. If it's not possible, focus on making one or two of the other days in the *Reflective* phase less hectic. The more time you can give people to change an appointment, a schedule, a deadline or an expectation, the more likely they will respond positively.

Apply your *Creative* phase abilities to any problems in your schedules by asking yourself how you could achieve the outcome you wish without being personally involved yourself, and see what solutions arise.

Creative phase

Day 25

Optimum Time for: Slowing down

When was the last time you took time to slow down? Modern culture drives us hard; we have to be available 24/7 and everything has the same top priority to be completed immediately. If we don't keep up we can feel guilty or frightened that we are under-achieving or that our job is at stake, or we can feel a sense of personal failure.

'Doing' and 'achieving' so often outweigh 'being' that we define our sense of self solely by the actions we take and the successes we create. We limit ourselves to wanting only our *Dynamic* phase aspect, running the risk that we'll lose out on the advantages of experiencing our inner depths. This creates stress because we can't naturally manage to maintain these levels of physical and mental energy and motivation. When we do finally stop or slow down, or a project ends, we can feel uncomfortable and lost; unable to simply be who we are because we haven't actually experienced who we are!

Accepting this Optimum Time forces us to prioritize our energy and actions, to be assertive in our scheduling, to set boundaries about what we will do, and to put a higher value on being who we are rather than on activity and achievements. When we do this we can still function productively in the busy world, but we do so from a perspective of inner calm and detachment. The effect of slowing down means that mental tasks and projects which would normally take five minutes might take a whole afternoon, and understanding or learning new structures or concepts may feel impossible. Our normal physical activities can become exhausting; the commute to work, the school run and the weekly shop can all seem overwhelming.

It can take a lot of courage to accept this aspect of our cycle and may involve some major re-organizing to enable ourselves to slow down. The rewards however are a break from the fast-lane, a reduction in stress, a more balanced perspective of what's important, creative inspiration, inner calm and acceptance, and the ability to re-enter the fast lane with renewed enthusiasm, personal strength and determination. On a long journey everyone needs comfort breaks every so often!

Well-being action: Allowing your Body to Slow down

Slow down! Your body needs it and so does your mind. For the next few days of your cycle, start slowing down. Try to arrange an extra ten minutes sleep or relaxation time, and when walking develop a Mediterranean 'stroll' rather than a 'city dash'.

Take catnaps during the day. The body's cycle of concentration lasts 90 minutes, so a quick ten minute 'time out' can help you to restore your energies.

Goal action: Being Realistic

You are going to get frustrated and stressed if you expect too much of yourself in the next few days. Be realistic in what you can achieve and don't criticize yourself if you can't maintain your usual high level of activity. You may find that your mental abilities will be reduced, making some tasks harder and therefore frustrating. Being aware of what you can do and keeping realistic will help, as well as reminding yourself that you have other talents and abilities in this phase which you can use.

Work enhancement action: Allocating more time

Allocate more time than you would normally allow to any tasks you have to do today. You may find that you think slower and are physically slower, so doing tasks takes longer. If you are unable to avoid a hectic and demanding day, try to balance it with more relaxation time in the evening or during the following day. If you are self-employed and are charging hourly for your work, you will need to take this into consideration. Remember that you will get more achieved in the *Dynamic* phase.

Just for today, try appreciating your sense of slowing down. Watch everyone else running around frantic and stressed, and appreciate that as you have determined your work priorities and allocated more time to your schedules there is no need to lose your sense of inner calm.

Creative phase

Day 26

Optimum Time for: Clearing the Decks

During the *Creative* phase we can experience explosive emotional feelings, pent up physical energy, frustration and intolerance. The more we try to repress or restrict these feelings the more likely they are to slip through unexpectedly. The smallest event can trigger the release of a cascade of emotions and feelings out of proportion to the circumstances.

These feelings and impulses are not negative; they are an indicator of a need for change, and are a powerful and positive force for transformation if we focus them in the right direction. Without giving these energies application and the opportunity to flow, we can often feel at the mercy of overwhelming forces outside of our control. Many women instinctively release their *Creative* phase feelings safely in frantic tidying and spring-cleaning. The underlying desire behind the *Creative* phase is 'to create', and our sense of intolerance and frustration are feelings which naturally cut away at the superfluous and stagnant to create space for something new to develop.

This makes the *Creative* phase the Optimum Time to look at our environment, projects, goals, and work, and to clear out things we no longer need and aspects that no longer work or which are unproductive. It's the opportunity for us to prune back to allow new growth to occur.

By taking the *Creative* phase opportunity to release our feelings and emotions constructively, we also gain the added advantage of carrying a lighter load of emotional baggage into the next month.

Well-being action: Clearing Emotionally

Look around your living environment and listen to your feelings. What feels annoying, messy, dirty or in need of a good clean? Now is the time to start cleaning and clearing.

Allow any feelings of frustration, physical tension, intolerance and stress flow through you as you clean. These feelings may be linked to past events, actions and relationships, and can generate images and conversations in your mind. The need to clean and clear externally originates from a strong inner need for emotional release and for self-acceptance, forgiveness and letting go.

Keep your focus on your cleaning and give the emotions permission to be there. It can be hard to allow them freedom, but you have a wonderful and powerful opportunity to accept your past self, to forgive, and to love yourself. Ask yourself, do you really want to carry this past emotional baggage into yet another month?

Goal action: Focusing your Energy

This is the Optimum Time to clear out approaches and action plans which are not working for you.

What hasn't worked since this time last month? Look back at the action list you made in the *Dynamic* phase, and ask yourself which actions still feel important enough to do? Which goals haven't been met, what approaches aren't working and need changing?

Focus your energies on what's important. What tasks do you want to take through to the next month? What will you leave behind? Make a new list to review in the *Reflective* phase.

Work Enhancement action: Clearing Out

Look around at your work environment and ask yourself which areas need more organization, tidying or cleaning. What needs sorting out? Now is the time to do something about it!

A warning!

In this phase there's a tendency to get caught up in the whirlwind of frantic clearing, and throw away things which could still be useful. To be safe, keep to one side a pile of things that may be needed in the future, preferably somewhere out of sight. Go back to this pile in your *Dynamic* phase when you will have more clarity about whether it will be needed.

This is also a good time to identify and clear out aspects of projects which are no longer productive or effective. Use your *Creative* phase abilities to identify and clear stagnant areas, along with seeding your subconscious to create new ideas for the way ahead. Don't start anything new just yet, or fix anything now, you'll do that in the *Dynamic* phases. Just for now acknowledge what is important or useful and clear away what isn't.

Creative phase

Day 27

Optimum Time for: Listening to our Inner Needs

For many of us the *Creative* phase, with its intense mood swings, out of control thoughts, and self-criticism, can seem a very harsh phase, and we often long for the hormones to change and for us to return back to 'normal' again. But if we only focus on wishing for this phase to end, we miss out on the important messages it gives us about our innermost feelings and needs.

Our self-critical and negative thoughts are messengers. They show us our lack of sense of self, of love and empowerment, created by our denying or straying away from our true needs during the previous three weeks. Our reaction to these attacking thoughts can include trying to sedate them by emotional eating and drinking, ignoring their message by 'fixing' ourselves and our circumstances, or believing them completely, creating feelings of self-hatred and depression.

Our negative feelings are the response to believing our critical thoughts about ourselves. The more painful the emotion, the more hurtful the content of the thought we believe. Our sense of self-empowerment creates our inner strength and inner wholeness, and any disruption in the *Creative* phase is telling us that we have lost touch with who and what we are.

When we disbelieve the lies we are thinking and listen for the truth underneath, we can rebuild our sense of self by focusing on and fulfilling our inner needs. With a stronger sense of self our critical thoughts become less powerful, and this will release our *Creative* phase energies and abilities for something much more positive.

Well-being action: Listening to your Needs

Give up one minute of your time to focus on yourself and ask "What do I need to do at the moment to fulfill my needs of self love?" Take a whole minute. The answer may be something really simple. Whatever it is, commit to doing it, as this will help enhance your sense of self by validating and meeting your real needs.

You can take as many one minutes for yourself as you need throughout the day. To help prevent next month's *Creative* phase being emotionally disruptive you may like to try this technique at least once a day throughout the next month.

Goal action: Focusing on Underlying Needs

Do not take action on any negative thoughts about yourself or your goal! This means **not creating multiple new goals** and taking action on them because you believe you'll feel happier once you have achieved them. If these new goals are really in tune with your true needs, you will obtain confirmation during the *Reflective* phase review and you can take positive action in the *Dynamic* phase. Focus instead on acknowledging and understanding the messages beneath any critical thoughts.

Work action: Taking Nothing Personally

Take nothing personally! Nothing your co-workers say about your work is personal to you; rather it is a statement of their own feelings and needs. Nothing you say to yourself about your work is actually true either; it is simply a reflection of how you feel and **your current unfulfilled needs**. Once your hormones change your view on work will change, so nothing is actually certain or 'true.'

Remember that the emotions of the *Creative* phase are not 'bad' and that you are not 'bad' for having them. They are simply a powerful message to help you re-create harmony and self-empowerment.

End of Creative phase summary

To help you assess your experiences during your *Creative* phase, you may like to answer the following questions.

1. How did you experience your *Creative* phase? In comparison to the *Expressive* phase, how did you feel?

Emotionally	
Mentally	
Physically	

2. On which days of the plan did you feel that the information and actions were in-tune with your personal experiences?
3. Which abilities did you find enhanced or easier in this phase compared to the previous one?
4. How did you practically apply your heightened abilities this month?
5. What are you planning to do with these *Creative* phase Optimum Time abilities next month?
6. What was the most surprising, intriguing or amazing thing you discovered about yourself in this phase?

Personalizing the plan

You can personalize the plan to suit your own cycle by choosing the actions which are in-tune with your Optimum Time abilities and listing them against your cycle date. You can repeat individual actions over a number of days.

Fill in the table below and see if you can plan some tasks for next month which will make the best use of your enhanced abilities.

Creative Phase		
My Optimum Time for:		
Cycle day number	Optimum Time actions	Planned task for next month

Reflective phase

Day 1

Optimum Time for: Meditation and Being

Welcome to the *Reflective* phase. This is the first day of menstruation, conventionally called day 1 of the menstrual cycle and the lowest tide in our flowing energies.

This phase offers us an opportunity to take a break from the driving power of our mind and personality, and it's a time when the body rests and restores itself.

We have a unique Optimum Time of peace and calm, detachment, passivity, and a chance to connect with ourselves and the world at a deeper level.

The first day of menstruation can be one of mixed experiences and emotions; it can include pain and other uncomfortable symptoms, gratefulness for the change in hormones which rescues us from the turmoil of the *Creative* phase, and perhaps sadness or relief at the lack of conception. For some women their entry into the *Reflective* phase can occur a few days before or after menstruation.

With the change to the *Reflective* phase we can experience better levels of mental clarity and structured thought processes, which creates our tendency to think that everything is over and to expect a return to our 'normal' life. However, refusing ourselves this time of physical, mental and emotional hibernation fights this phase's natural feelings of contentment and well-being.

The *Reflective* phase is one of lower physical energies, deep emotions and a natural meditative mental state. We need to accept this phase and to let go of our expectations of 'normal' to enjoy the abilities of meditation, reflection, commitment and deep inner knowing that this Optimum Time creates in our lives.

Well-being action: Meditation

In this phase you have a natural ability to meditate, and if you have found it difficult to meditate in the past or wish to try meditation for the first time, this is the Optimum Time to practice. Choose a method which appeals to you or simply stare out of a window, sit in a park or a garden, watch a river, or relax on a bed or sofa.

Accept that you have been given the opportunity to experience a deeper sense of life and connection which clears away the mental rubbish and allows you to feel what really matters in life. You will feel better and calmer if you can enjoy this time rather than fighting it.

Goal action: Letting go

Let go of all thoughts about goals, action plans and tasks, and simply do nothing.

Forget about achieving, and instead concentrate on the small things in life such as enjoying your lunch, the feel of sunshine, the sounds of the traffic, and the colors around you. This holiday from living in your head gives you the space to realize that there is more to life than future achievements. You have the opportunity to feel how good it is to be alive and part of something much bigger than your dreams

Work Enhancement action: Working with your Energies

Hopefully you have been able to plan ahead for today, and the next couple of days, to make them less hectic than normal. At work you may have a tendency to resist this phase of hibernation, but unrealistic expectations simply lead to feelings of frustration and stress. Be realistic about how much you can achieve, and focus on one thing at a time as your multi-tasking skills may be limited. Notice when in the day you lose energy so that you can make the most of the times when you do feel more alert.

If the days are hectic, keep your evenings free so you can relax and let your body restore its energies.

Reflective phase

Day 2

Optimum Time for: Getting in Touch with your Self

The *Reflective* phase is our Optimum Time for letting go and for leaving aside the need to make immediate changes to the world.

Unlike the *Creative* phase, where we try to create ourselves and our life path by seeking outside of ourselves, the *Reflective* phase turns us inwards to the awareness and wisdom beneath our everyday thoughts and desires, to our authentic or core self. This phase gives us the unique opportunity to touch base with ourselves, to experience who we truly are and to discover where our path to happiness lies.

Most of the time we live through masks; for example at work we may have a professional mask, with our friends another mask, and with our partner and family yet another. Each mask is a collection of thoughts we have about who and what we are, what we can do and what is appropriate behavior. Although masks are helpful in the multiple roles we need to play, we can lose contact with the real person beneath all these masks. Sometimes it's a case of 'will the real person please stand up?'

Each month the *Reflective* phase gives us the opportunity to return to our real self beneath our expectations and those of other people. For some women this can be quite a difficult experience, especially if their perception of who they are is built on achievement, success, job labels or social labels such as being a 'mother'. Removing the masks and discovering emptiness can be frightening, but it enables us to ask 'What is there in life which starts to fill this space?' By trying out different ideas we can connect with those things that create feelings of completeness and well-being. Sometimes this means we need to return to an image of ourselves from the past or to activities that we used to do. This is not a step backwards, but more a realization of how far we have moved from our authentic self and its life path, and a commitment to getting our lives back on track.

Well-being action: Dropping the Baggage

You may find that some events during the month have created uncomfortable emotional baggage. Touching base with your authentic self at this time gives you the opportunity to let this baggage go and to create a fresh new image of yourself for the month ahead.

Take time today to simply relax and feel the well-being, self acceptance and connectedness which naturally underlie the *Reflective* phase. While centered in these feelings, review your emotions and the events that generated them. Ask yourself 'Can I be bothered with this emotion?', 'Can I be bothered with this past response/event?', and 'Can I be bothered to carry my reaction into the next month?' Your natural 'whatever' attitude at this time will help you to drop your emotional baggage.

Goal action: Rediscovering Fulfillment

Ask yourself 'What would bring me feelings of fulfillment and completeness?', 'What have I lost which I feel needs to be restored?' and 'What is important to me?'

Don't try to analyze the questions or yourself; simply relax and let yourself be guided by your feelings. Sometimes the answer can seem daunting, but when the feelings behind a change are positive and strong they give you the strength and commitment to make the change.

Over the next few days, daydream about your responses to these questions and the actions the answers are requesting. This will allow your consciousness to get used to any unsettling ideas and build the commitment you need to make the first steps in the month ahead.

Work Enhancement action: Being True to Yourself

Now is the time to take a realistic look at your work 'mask'. Does how you behave and what you do at work align with your authentic self? What fresh, new and truer image of yourself could you take into the next month?

Take a spare moment to make a list of all your core values and the things which bring you joy and happiness in both your home and working life. Try not to limit, analyze, or justify the list. Don't take any action on the list contents, or make any commitments or promises to yourself yet; simply enjoy this reflection of who you are at this moment.

If you have a list from last month, notice what has changed and what has remained the same.

Reflective phase

Day 3

Optimum Time for: Discovering the Real Priorities

The *Reflective* phase has better mental skills and clarity than the *Creative* phase, but with limited physical energy and motivation we need to focus this energy on our highest priorities.

We all carry an internal list of 'shoulds' which has developed out of the expectations of our family, our society, and our working environment, on what we have to do to be accepted, loved, to have power and to be safe. Our 'shoulds' are created out of the stories that people tell us and the stories we tell ourselves.

The word 'should' often comes attached with emotions of guilt, and we can carry guilt from unmet expectations in the past as well as adding to the emotional baggage every month with our list of things to do.

The *Reflective* phase attitude of not 'being bothered' about things is helpful for realizing that our 'shoulds' are based on others' demands on us, and this empowers us to release these expectations. When we do this we free ourselves of guilt and experience greater freedom of choice.

The *Reflective* phase is the Optimum Time to revisit our list of required actions, look at the expectations we have about our life, work and goals, and find out what is really important to us. We can ask ourselves why we're using the word 'should' rather than 'could', and look at the fears associated with the unachieved outcome and our resistance to doing the task. Releasing our 'shoulds' changes our perception for the month ahead to an empowering internal list of 'coulds'. We give ourselves a free and unburdened choice of actions to take.

Well-being action: Changing 'Shoulds' into 'Coulds'

We build our internal list of 'shoulds' from other people's stories on how the world needs to be for them to feel loved and safe. Which of your 'shoulds' are not your own? Whose story do you believe? How many of the 'shoulds' from childhood you are still carrying around? Change the word 'should' into 'could' in any thoughts or statements you make. The word 'could' gives you a choice to take action or not.

Goal action: Refining your Internal List

Write down your internal list of 'things to do'.

Put everything down, including childhood goals and unfulfilled dreams. Mark next to each action how long it has been on your mental and emotional list. Now mark next to each item whether you think it is a 'should'. Are there any actions on the list which you desperately want to do or really want done? Underline these. Take a big black marker pen and delete the 'shoulds' and… feel the emotional weight of all those 'shoulds' and their attached guilt disappear! Take no action towards your underlined list now. It will become the basis of your goal list for the next *Dynamic* phase.

Work action: Identifying Pressure Sources

Take a moment to review the pressures you feel on yourself at work. What makes you feel stressed or unhappy? Ask yourself, what are people's expectations of you and your work? Are these reasonable expectations given your job description, salary, schedules, training, skills and time available? Could you do your job better without carrying the pressure of other people's 'shoulds' into the next month? Can you identify the fear behind their expectations of you and perhaps alleviate it?

> # Reflective phase
>
> # Day 4

Optimum Time for: Letting Go of Resistance

The naturally low energy of the *Reflective* phase offers us the chance to let go of worries and concerns, simply because we don't have the energy to spare for them. When we stop resisting this phase and accept the slow down something wonderful happens. We experience a place of calm and well-being lying beneath our everyday noisy thoughts. Within this inner space lie feelings of acceptance, wholeness and a deep sense that everything is and will be okay. Unfortunately modern society doesn't easily give us the opportunity to let go and relax in this phase, and it's our need to meet society's expectations which increases our resistance to the *Reflective* phase.

To resist comes automatically to most of us. Built on layers of thoughts about our safety, we resist and fight anything which seems to threaten it. The more we resist, the more inflexible we become and the further our perspective moves from the reality of the situations we find ourselves faced with. When we realize that surrendering to the Reflective phase actively brings empowerment, control, strength and well-being, we are more likely to let go of any resistance to slowing down.

The wonderful opportunity the *Reflective* phase gives us is to feel that life is just fine the way it is at this moment. It grounds us in the present, helping us to let go of our future expectations and past memories. It is the Optimum Time for reflecting on current worries and anxieties, as our natural connection with our inner assurance enables us to discover how unreal they are and to trust the process of life. We often lose this connection amid the bustle of the rest of the month, but for now we have the amazing option to enjoy the beautiful sensation of everything being okay just the way it is.

Well-being action: Let Go of Expectations

Are you resisting your *Reflective* phase? Can you, for a few days each month, simply let go of your expectations, and gracefully accept that things will need to be put aside, dropped or take a little longer?

Why do you think you are resisting this opportunity to slow down and connect with a deeper aspect of yourself? Just for today slow right down. Allow nothing to really matter, and notice how your body relaxes in response and your feelings of happiness increase. Throughout the day take a little time to notice your breath. Notice how good it feels when the body receives the air it needs, and how good it feels when it exhales the air it doesn't. Focus on these good feelings and the inner experience of assurance it generates.

Goal action: Discovering your Resistance

When we experience discomfort with anything, we are resisting something. Think about your goals and your actions towards them over the past month and notice when and where you have felt emotional, mental or physical stress. These sensations tell you that you are resisting the situation.

It may be that your goals and actions are not in tune with your authentic self, your needs at the time, or that you are trying to force reality to go the way you want rather than accepting it the way it really is.

Which areas do you feel this applies to and which areas seem to be flowing easily with minimal effort?

Acknowledging that your true self is resisting the way the mind is forcing it to go is the first step toward letting go and reviewing your goals.

Work action: Taking a New Direction

Think about areas where you feel you are putting in a lot of effort, time or money, and not seeing positive outcomes or returns.

Are you putting your energies in the right direction or resisting the situation and fighting to get your own way?

Could you let go of your current approach and try another direction to achieve the positive results you want?

Reflective phase

Day 5

Optimum Time for: Reviewing

The *Reflective* phase is the Optimum Time to review our lives and goals to see whether they are still in keeping with what we want to achieve, and whether we still have the original incentive and enthusiasm to make things happen.

In the *Reflective* phase, reviewing is not an analytical process but one which is guided by the natural connection we have at this time to our deeper inner levels. 'Reviewing' is more like meditation or reflection, with an emphasis on our feelings and intuitions.

During the *Creative* phase we can experience intense revelations or strong urges to cut loose on certain situations, activities or people – but we should leave taking action until we have gone through the Reflective phase. This is the time to hold the idea in our minds and to test it out on our feelings of 'rightness' and well-being. We need to ask ourselves if it feels right to make an ending and to create something new, or whether we can view the situation in an impersonal way and let it go with the past month. The situation may actually be okay but just needs improving in certain areas.

The *Reflective* phase offers us the opportunity to review situations and to reflect on our feelings about them before we make a commitment to action.

Cutting things free in the *Reflective* phase happens at a deep level and has the potential to make a powerful and positive change on our lives. Letting go with the inner knowledge that it's 'the right thing to do' helps to both support us against mental pressure when the mind starts to become more analytical and questioning in the *Dynamic* phase and to protect us from the pressure of other people's views.

The process of reviewing in the *Reflective* phase also opens us to deep-level insights and ideas about situations. Simply by acknowledging and being with a problem or issue we open a door for new perceptions to flow through.

Well-being action: Reflecting on Issues

Choose a single issue which has been causing you discomfort, and acknowledge its effect on you and your life. Ask yourself if you need to let something go; for example a memory, an emotional reaction, a relationship, an expectation, a disappointment, an attitude, a judgment or criticism, or even a dream. Ask yourself if the situation actually feels okay but needs improving in certain areas. Allow yourself to reflect on your issue as well as on these questions and your answers throughout the day.

If you feel it's time to let go, test it against your feelings of 'rightness', and then commit to taking positive action next month in the most appropriate phases.

Goal action: Checking your Progress

Look at your goals and action plan from last month, or write down the wish list you have been carrying in your head. Goals are simply places we aim for, and during the journey towards them we often discover new things we wish to do or new aspects of ourselves we wish to explore. Reviewing is simply checking your progress and whether you are still traveling in the right direction.

This is the Optimum Time to reflect on whether you wish to spend the next month traveling towards the goals you have set. Does it feel exciting to commit time and effort next month to making your goal happen, or does it no longer feel worth it? Where does your enthusiasm and happiness lie?

Do you have too many diverse goals which dilute your energies? Choose or re-affirm one main over-riding goal, however wild and out of reach it you may think it is.

Work Enhancement action: Getting an Overview

Use this invaluable Optimum Time for reviewing, to look over work projects, task lists, structures and schedules, or the diary for the month ahead. Remember, you're not trying to analyze anything – leave that to the *Dynamic* phase. You are trying to get an overview 'feel' of what feels right and good.

Your intuition will point out areas which don't feel 'right'. At the time you may not intellectually understand the reasons behind your feelings, but your subconscious will be recognizing patterns you may be missing consciously. Trust your intuition, and give it time over the next few days to come up with the reasons. There will be an answer to 'why', but it may take a little time for it to take form.

Reflective phase

Day 6

Optimum Time for: Setting up for the Dynamic Phase

The *Dynamic* phase will be our Optimum Time for taking the inspiration, ideas and inner knowing from the *Creative* and *Reflective* phases and putting them into dynamic action. It's our Optimum Time for getting things done and making plans, which makes it the ideal starting point for the new month.

The energies and abilities of the *Reflective* phase gradually transform into those of the *Dynamic* phase, and to make best use of these new energies we need to decide where we are going to focus our newly restored and rejuvenated energies and abilities.

As we emerge from the hibernation of the *Reflective* phase, our physical energies start to increase; we need less sleep and have more stamina. Mentally we pay more attention to the outer world, and we are renewed with greater clarity and enthusiasm for the direction and actions we want to take.

With better memory and processing power it's the Optimum Time to learn something new, to try new experiences, to build structure and plan the steps to our dreams.

We not only have the ability to enthuse about the bigger picture but also to plan the smaller steps to create it. Our confidence will also increase during the *Dynamic* phase, and once again our self belief tells us we can do and achieve anything we put our minds to. The *Dynamic* phase is a wonderful opportunity to start afresh, and with the creativity and clearing out of the *Creative* phase and the reviewing of the *Reflective* phase, we are now in the best position to move forward on the journey towards our goals and dreams.

Well-being action: Choosing Adventures

What could you do in the next week that's adventurous, fun, new and exciting, and which you could use the Dynamic phase organizing skills to make happen? Think outside the box. Think of something you've always wanted to try but lacked the self-confidence to do. If you can't do it this month, start organizing it for next month.

Also reflect on what you'd really like to do with all this new energy coming to you. You may want to start a new healthy diet and fitness regime, take on a new project, start a course or learn a new skill.

Goal action: Targeting action

Start thinking about your goals and the actions you need to take towards them in the month ahead. The *Dynamic* phase is going to give you the energy and clarity to work out all the details and create the structure and schedules you'll need to achieve them, so it's important that you have a clear idea of where and how you want to apply these abilities. Use your insights from this *Reflective* phase to help you keep focused on your highest priorities.

Work action: Focusing your Energies

The *Dynamic* phase is going to offer you extra mental clarity, good multi-tasking skills and the ability to focus and concentrate for longer. This is obviously the time to catch up on the tasks which you put on hold during the *Reflective* phase, so it can be useful to put together a list of tasks and to prioritize each item.

Reflect on areas which you feel need more organization and structure, more effective time management, or more information on a subject, before you take action. The analytical abilities of the *Dynamic* phase are ideal for solving problems and dealing with detail. Be aware that in the *Dynamic* phase there will be the tendency to become too achievement and work-orientated. As you enter this phase keep in mind that although you can catch up and achieve a lot at work it is important not to do it at the expense of your work /life balance.

End of Reflective phase summary

To help you assess your experiences during your *Reflective* phase, you may like to answer the following questions.

1. How did you experience your *Reflective* phase? In comparison to the *Creative* phase, how did you feel?

Emotionally	
Mentally	
Physically	

2. On which days of the plan did you feel that the information and actions were in-tune with your personal experiences?
3. Which abilities did you find enhanced or easier in this phase compared to the previous one?
4. How did you practically apply your heightened abilities this month?
5. What are you planning to do with these *Reflective* phase Optimum Time abilities next month?
6. What was the most surprising, intriguing or amazing thing you discovered about yourself in this phase?

Personalizing the plan

You can personalize the plan to suit your own cycle by choosing the actions which are in-tune with your Optimum Time abilities and listing them against your cycle date. You can repeat individual actions over a number of days.

Fill in the table below and see if you can plan some tasks for next month which will make the best use of your enhanced abilities.

Reflective Phase		
My Optimum Time for:		
Cycle day number	Optimum Time actions	Planned task for next month

Chapter 10

Done the plan, so what's next?

The Optimized Woman Daily Plan is a map which begins a journey of self exploration and discovery. Working with the plan changes our view of ourselves, regardless of how many or how few of the daily actions we actively implement

> "Every cycle is such a discovery!! I love it. And the more conscious I become of it, the more intense I seem to live it." Sophia, Doula and Workshop Facilitator, Spain.

in our lives. Sometimes just knowing that there is a different perspective is enough to alter the way we look at things. Sometimes just being given permission to act in tune with our authentic self is enough to change our lives.

The plan helps us to view our cycles in a new light, as a positive resource of Optimum Times and abilities which we can apply to many different areas of our lives.

Our approach to the various phases of our cycle can become one of excitement and anticipation at experiencing, exploring and applying these enhanced abilities.

The plan has guided us into the territory of our own unique cycles, so now we need to take the next step and explore and map out this new and exciting landscape. To do this we need to understand the shape and form of the land, the challenges and opportunities which are distinct to ourselves.

Moving from linear to cyclic awareness

By now you will have taken the results from the phase summary sheets and looked at your diary to mark in the phases and perhaps the Optimum Time skills for the month ahead. The problem with a diary is that it represents a linear concept of time, and by using it to record our cycles to plan our time we strengthen the view that our cycles are simply a repeating sequence rather than a repeating rotation.

To help us to reinforce our awareness of our cyclic nature and abilities we can record our Optimum Time and enhanced skill sets on a series of circular diagrams or Cycle Dials similar to those suggested in *The Wise Wound* by Penelope Shuttle and Peter Redgrove. The advantage of a Cycle Dial over an ordinary diary is the ability to quickly compare two or more months at a glance, enabling us to discover more easily the patterns behind our abilities and their Optimum Times.

Creating a Cycle Dial

A Cycle Dial is a circular diary for one menstrual cycle. To create a Cycle Dial we simply draw a circle on a sheet of paper and subdivide it into radial sections where each section represents a day in the cycle. Additional blank days are included in case the cycle for the month is longer than expected (see Figure 4). Although the example dial is based on a 28 day cycle, your cycle may be longer or shorter than this.

The circle is then divided into three concentric rings, with the outer ring used for recording the 'day number' of the cycle. The first day of menstruation is referred to as 'day 1' of the cycle because it's the easiest day to identify. We have seen in the plan that the real physical, mental and emotional start of the cycle begins with the increase in energy accompanying the start of the *Dynamic* phase around day 7.

As the entry into the *Dynamic* phase is not always on the same day however, it can be useful to start each Cycle Dial on the first day of menstruation, i.e. day 1. **Remember that this is not the start of the new energy cycle which begins with the start of the *Dynamic* phase**.

The middle ring is for the calendar date, and it's helpful to fill in these dates in advance. The inner ring is used for recording a few key descriptive words.

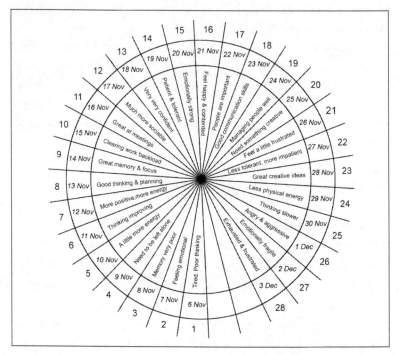

Figure 4 Example of a completed dial

A blank Cycle Dial is supplied in Appendix 2 for copying and enlarging for personal use. A downloadable version is also available from **www.optimizedwoman.com**.

Creating an 'Overview Dial'

An Overview Dial is our own map of the landscape of our cycle. It can be used to help us plan the month ahead by giving us a summary of our cycle at a glance.

To make an Overview Dial, take your notes from the 'personalizing the plan' summary information for each phase, with its relevant cycle day number. Write this information on a blank dial, leaving the calendar date empty.

If you wish, color the days with specific enhanced abilities to emphasize your Optimum Times. You now have an Overview Dial which is an invaluable tool for planning the month ahead.

Our Overview Dial needs to be used with the understanding that our cycles can be changeable and that outside influences can have an impact.

Our enhanced skills will sometimes vary on the days they appear, so we still need to be alert to our changes as and when they occur and to act on them accordingly. With this in mind we can use the dial to help us plan actions to coincide with our Optimum Times in the month ahead.

Creating a 'Planning Dial'

> **The Planning Dial is probably one of the simplest and most powerful tools you will encounter to create the life, success, fulfillment and well-being you want.**

A Planning Dial is simply a circular way of planning the month ahead based on our Optimized Times and associated skills. Create a blank dial for the month ahead with your cycle day numbers and calendar dates in place. Then, in your *Dynamic* phase, and with reference to your 'to do' list and Overview Dial, allocate activities to particular days on

"I plan my month according to my cycle: public engagements are scheduled around my ovulation, which is my most outgoing time of the month. Writing, planning and material-gathering are saved for menstruation, the most introverted time of the month for me." DeAnna, Speaker, Educator and Trainer, USA.

the dial.

Unlike a diary where you may have to flick through different pages, the dial provides you with the month's plan of action at a glance.

Create as many Planning Dials as you like. You can have individual ones for specific projects, or more general ones for work, self-development and goal achievement.

For example, for work you can use the Planning Dial to plan:

- Specific actions
- Relaxed days
- Catch-up days
- Creative days
- Meetings and presentations
- Researching and learning days
- Networking days
- Problem identification and blue-sky thinking days
- Starting, supporting, and reviewing projects days
- Deadlines

When using your cycles for personal life-coaching you can use a Planning Dial to plan for the activities you've outlined in your monthly action plan.

Use the dial to:

- Plan a *Reflective* phase day as a review day
- Mark a *Dynamic* day as an action planning day
- Plan actions in tune with your Optimum Times
- Plan research and networking days

You can also use the Planning Dial to make best use of your Optimum Times to help your personal life and self-development.

Use it to organize:

- Social commitments to coincide with energetic, outgoing and nurturing times
- Health and fitness regimes, taking into account of low energy times and adjust expectations accordingly
- 'Me' times to relax, nurture, reflect and touch base
- A day for personal accounts, bill paying, and clearing the 'to do' list
- New projects - this can be anything ranging from home decorating to a taking a class to starting a business
- Alone time to reflect, to understand core issues and to release emotions, fears and anxieties
- The opportunity and tools to release creativity and to express yourself
- Time for heart-to-heart discussions, relationships and family

The Planning Dial also gives us the opportunity to make sure that we meet the mental, emotional and creative needs of each of the four phases by planning supportive activities in tune with each phase. Revisit *Chapters 4 to 7* for ideas and strategies to use with the Planning Dial, and look at the tables in *Chapter 11* for a summary of skills and aptitudes.

By changing how we view ourselves and our lives, and planning to actively live in tune with our cycles, we build our feelings of empowerment, success and, most importantly, of self-acceptance, love and happiness.

If we plan, and take action on only one thing in an Optimum Time, we will achieve more, or reach a higher level of performance, than we would have otherwise.

Taking the next step

The plan is designed as a starting point, and the next step is to go that bit deeper into the variety of changes we can experience during the month. During the plan you will have experienced changes in yourself not covered by the plan. You may have observed fluctuations in your sexual desires and changes in your emotional and relationship needs, spirituality, dreams, and food cravings.

Appendix 1 has tables outlining some of the changes we may experience during the month. Some of them will be immediately familiar, and some will seem strange. Don't be put off by the lists; we don't need to record everything, but a wider variety of observations can help us to better understand our changes.

Some women like to keep a journal and use summary keywords on their Cycle Dials.

If record-keeping doesn't appeal or life is just too hectic for yet another thing to do, a quick alternative is to give numerical values to our obser-

> "(*Day 23. Creative phase*) Very tired, need for more sleep. Attention span and focus bad 2/10 (no brain at all!!)"
> Déborah, Fashion House Assistant Stylist, France.

vations; for example, if we are noting our physical stamina we could simply record 4 / 10 on a low day.

The more we understand our Optimum Times and their enhanced abilities, the more we are able to create a life for ourselves which inherently brings happiness and well-being.

The challenge is to live our cyclic nature in a world which doesn't support it. It is possible, it just takes a bit of planning, and the rewards outweigh the challenges.

For me, understanding my cycle showed me skills I didn't know I had, and I've been able to use them successfully because I was prepared to see that one week, once a month, was an opportunity and not a failure to be consistent throughout the month.

She who dares wins!

> **Rather than a failure to be consistent, one week of skills once a month is an opportunity for success.**

The last and final step in 'What's next?' is to ask ourselves how we share this information about our cycles with the men in our lives.

When I gave talks on my book, *Red Moon: Understanding and using the gifts of the menstrual cycle*, I was amazed and pleased at the number of men in the audience. Some were therapists, but most were men who wanted to understand the women in their lives and to learn how to get along with them better. The problem most men have is; if we don't understand how we work, how are they supposed to know?

> **If women don't understand who they are and how they work, how are men supposed to know?!**

The key to any relationship is communication, and we need to communicate our experiences and understanding of our own unique Optimum Times.

Obviously in a working environment it can feel awkward and inappropriate to talk to male colleagues about our menstrual cycle. The subject has public taboos and it can take a strong woman to manage the jokes, the derogative terms and comments, put-downs, the sweeping generalizations and the negative associations. We can, however, help men to understand our changing abilities during our menstrual cycle and encourage our employers to work with our strengths, simply by using the term 'Optimum Time'. Saying that this week or next week will be an 'optimum time' for certain tasks gives strong guidance to male colleagues on what to expect from us. Whether we explain the basis of our Optimum Times or not will depend on our relationship with our colleagues.

One of the comments I received again and again after writing *Red Moon* was 'I wish my husband would read this book'. If you have a man who is interested, and who will sit and read a book on the menstrual cycle from start to finish, then hand this over. A friend's husband sat reading *Red Moon* in biker leathers on the London Underground on his way to work each morning. You can imagine the looks he received!

Most men, I expect, will simply want a summary containing 'what to expect' and 'what to do', and I have provided this in *Chapter 11*. My husband has always wanted a colored indicator on my forehead telling him which phase I am in. We compromised on a series of colored fridge magnets. Obviously we can't give our partners the definite criteria they would like or fix rules on what will work with us and what won't, so it's still important for us to share our experiences and give them guidelines.

Sharing experiences is however a two-way process; we also need to listen to our partner's feelings about who we are and how we behave in our different phases and to find ways to both meet our needs and support our partner's needs. If we think about it, our partner is essentially living with four different women in one body.

Men are living with four women in one body!

When we do bring our Optimum Times into our relationships with men, we create a win-win situation. By giving work colleagues guidelines on our Optimum Times for tasks, they begin to tailor work to fit around these times because of the heightened creativity, productivity and skill sets we offer.

In our personal relationships, we are more able to express who we are and what we need, enabling men to feel confident about meeting those needs without the fear of getting things wrong or of rejection.

> "I was surprised that my partner is very interested in it (*Optimium Times*) too. This is going to help him understand me better. It's win win!!"
> Wendy, Marketing Director, Canada.

Chapter 10 Summary

- Using a circular record dial or *Cycle Dial* enables us to compare months more easily.
- A Cycle Dial helps us to realize that we are cyclic in nature.
- We can create a single dial as a summary overview of our Optimum Times skills and abilities and use it as a tool for planning activities in the month ahead.
- When we apply a skill or ability in its Optimum Time, we reach a level of productivity, insight or excellence that we would otherwise miss.
- We can experience a wide range of Optimum Time abilities. Keeping a more detailed record enables us to discover the full potential our cycle offers us.
- A skill for one week is not 'being inconsistent', but is an opportunity to explore, develop and succeed in new areas.
- Men need to know about our Optimum Times to prevent false expectations and generalizations about our skills and abilities.
- Using the term 'Optimum Times' in the workplace helps men to understand the concept, even if it's inappropriate to mention the menstrual cycle.
- We need to share our experiences of our Optimum Times with our partners and to listen to their needs in relation to those experiences.
- **It is necessary to tell partners which phase we are in**.

Chapter 11

What men need to know

First of all, congratulations for starting this chapter! I'm guessing that you have a female partner or work with women. I'm also guessing that you have been given this chapter to read. Don't worry – I will make this quick and straightforward.

In this section I'm going to briefly summarize the main points you need to know on how women work, and provide you with some suggestions on how to apply this information. Although it won't explain every woman, it will give you a few keys to what's happening in a lot of women.

Why women don't think and behave like men

The bad news is that women are not like men, so men need some strategies for approaching them. The key to understanding women is to realize that they are not

> "Why can't a woman be more like a man?" Professor Henry Higgins from the musical 'My Fair Lady'.

consistent in their abilities, skills and thought processes from week to week. This probably doesn't come as any great revelation; however, if you understand that women are consistent on a monthly basis, then there is a level of predictability.

The '4 in 1' Woman

Imagine that you have four different women, one a week for a month. Each woman has slightly different abilities and ways of perceiving the world. Your approach to each woman would naturally be slightly different, and your expectations of each woman would be different as well.

Now imagine that these four women all look alike and you have the basis for understanding women and their menstrual cycles. Each woman is at least four different women in one!

Every woman is at least four different women in one!

Each month women go through four phases in their menstrual cycles which gives them access to different skills and abilities.

This doesn't mean that women are unreliable or inconsistent; rather that they have access to a wide range of enhanced or heightened abilities and approaches on a repeating monthly basis. Women have a powerful skill set that is often underused because their skills are seen as erratic.

Living and working with the '4 in 1' woman means that men need to change their expectations on how they should approach and work with women.

> Never trust something that bleeds for seven days and doesn't die!" Mr Garrison from *South Park* television program.

The good news is that if you align your approach to a woman's heightened skills and way of thinking, you are not only more likely to be well received but you will also be given surprising levels of action, commitment, problem solving, creativity, support or understanding in response.

If you align your approach to a woman's Optimum Time skills and way of thinking, you are more likely to receive a positive response.

So what are the Optimum Times?

These are groups of days during the month where women display heightened skill sets. These skills range from mental skills such as multi-tasking, analysis, structured and creative thinking, to emotional skills such as empathy, networking and team support, and physical skills such as stamina, strength and co-ordination.

The cycle can be divided into four Optimum Times, each of which is roughly a week long, although this will vary between women. I have called these Optimum Times the *Dynamic* phase, the *Expressive* phase, the *Creative* phase and the *Reflective* phase, and they correspond to the pre-ovulation, the ovulation, the premenstrual and the menstrual phases of a woman's cycle in turn.

What you need to know about women

To approach women in-tune with their Optimum Times, you obviously need to understand what many women experience during these times. Then to make the most of these enhanced abilities and skills you also need to know what type of actions and tasks women will excel at during these times.

Finally, and probably the most important, you also need to know how to adapt your approach in response to the Optimum Times, and to know how to guess which phase a woman is in.

Table 11.1 Women's Optimum Times and their skills and aptitudes

Cycle phase	Optimum Time skills and aptitudes
Dynamic phase Approximately days 7 – 13	Concentration, memory recall, planning, attention to detail, structured and logical thinking, achievement focused, independent action, and self motivated. Excellent physical stamina and strength.
Expressive phase Approximately days 14 – 20	People-focused, effective communication, empathy, team player, networking, sales, teaching, altruistic approach, support, productive, flexible, emotionally strong. Good physical, mental and emotional strength and stamina.
Creative phase Approximately days 21 – 28	Critical analysis, problem solving, independent action, control, creative, intuitive, enthusiasm fired motivation, focused on change and problems. Gradual decrease in mental and physical energy, and an increase in emotional sensitivity. Peaks of high creativity and also of frustration.
Reflective phase Approximately days 1 – 6	Impartial reviewing, overview approach, detachment from outcomes, letting go,

	forgiving, core beliefs important, creative reflection, intuitive understanding, feelings orientated. Low mental and physical energies.

Remember that women can have all these abilities throughout the month; the Optimum Times are simply groups of days where particular skills and aptitudes are heightened.

Table 11.2 Women's Optimum Time actions

Cycle phase	Optimum Time actions
Dynamic phase Approximately days 7 – 13	**A good time for:** • Logic tasks and problem solving • Learning • Planning • Detailed report writing • Understanding and structuring complex information • Starting projects **Not a good time for:** • Summary or brief reports • A casual attitude • Joint projects • An empathic approach
Expressive phase Approximately days 14 – 20	**A good time for:** • Caring • Supporting people and projects • Discussing feelings and relationship problems

	• Joint projects
	• Leadership roles
	• Creating emotionally centered approaches
	• Building relationships
	Not a good time for:
	• Analysis and technical detail
	• Emotional detachment
	• Independent action
	• Motivation through material outcomes
Creative phase Approximately days 21 – 28	**A good time for:** • Critical analysis • Identification of problems • Taking independent action • Creative input and solutions • Clearing and sorting • Reorganizing • Focusing on the outcome • Being a driving force • Controlling situations or projects **Not a good time for:** • Heart to heart discussions • Negotiations • Inactivity • Detailed, precise work • Logical reasoning
Reflective phase Approximately days 1 – 6	**A good time for:** • Reviewing projects and relationships • Focus on core principles • Appraising feedback • Committing to decisions and changes

	• Assessing personal life goals and direction
	• Creative reflection
	• Intuitive insight
	Not a good time for:
	• Physical stamina
	• Learning and memory skills
	• Concentration
	• Working additional hours
	• Material motivation

Getting the Best from Women

The way to get the best from women is to:

- Match tasks to their Optimum Times.
- Alter your communication and approach to tie-in with their skills and abilities.

If you use an emotional approach to ask a woman for something when she's in her Optimum Time for details and logic, your request may be rejected, ignored or given a very low priority. If, however, you alter your approach and give structured reasons, not only are you more likely to be given a high priority but you may also receive detailed results, productivity and timescales well beyond your expectations.

Table 11.3 Methods of approaching women during their Optimum Times

Cycle phase	Optimum Time approaches
Dynamic phase Approximately days and 7 – 13	• Offer new projects. • Give logical reasons for what you want, make your request or requirement seem to coincide with her goals. • Be seen to give support to her 'causes' but allow her the space to take the initiative and work on her own. • Acknowledge her self-motivation, and use her attention to detail for planning. • Keep non-task communication for the following week.
Expressive phase Approximately days 14 – 20	• Suggest networking or socializing. • Provide projects which involve caring or nurturing, or working as a team towards a joint goal. • Provide positive validation. • Give altruistic or people-oriented reasons for what you want, and ask for what you want directly. • Share your feelings and use emotional words in communications.
Creative phase Approximately days 21 – 28	• Be flexible and prioritize tasks. • Offer subjects for break-through ideas. • Motivate through enthusiasm and creativity, and use undemanding language.

	• Offer support or give her independence as required. • Focus her critical judgment skills away from you. • Understand that her 'problems' do not need to be solved immediately by you, but some action needs to be taken.
Reflective phase Approximately days 1 – 6	•Accept that this is a low energy week and schedule tasks to coincide with her renewed energies in the following week. •Introduce any challenging new ideas or changes for her to process, and to commitment to. •Ask what is really important to her. •Understand that groundbreaking insight is still there, it may just take a couple of days to come through. •Allow 'down' time and personal space, and reduce pressure for immediate results.

How Can a Man Tell which Optimum Time a Woman is in?

This is a tricky question to answer as many women are unaware of their cyclic abilities. They often ignore or suppress their cycle's effects to fit in with work and life expectations. The key however is communication and observation.

A simple method is to try out different approaches based on the lists above. You may have to ask four times in four different ways, but the tactic which provides a positive response will give you an indication of the Optimum Time.

For example, if you want a report written, one approach would be to offer four different slants to see which idea is met with confidence and enthusiasm. Options could be to suggest; she collates and structures a list of detailed observations and information (*Dynamic* phase), she takes a people-orientated focus (*Expressive* phase), she uses the report to identify problems and creative solutions (*Creative* phase), or she creates a general overview report focusing on company core values (*Reflective* phase).

Another way to identify the Optimum Time is to notice the language a woman uses and the tasks she is excited or enthusiastic about.

If she has created a long detailed list of things for you to do, the chances are she is in her *Dynamic* phase. If she has created a long detailed list of things which are wrong (including you) and an equally long list of things for you to do to put them right, the chances are she is in her *Creative* phase!

Although women's physical energy levels may seem to be a good indicator of the Optimum Times, unfortunately many women use extra caffeine to over-ride the body's need to slow down in the *Creative* and *Reflective* phases.

A word of warning! Using the information in this chapter in a way which could be interpreted as defining, belittling, or dismissive, will not earn you a positive response or respect! Women dislike men using the menstrual cycle as a joke or as a definitive reason or excuse for female behavior.

The abilities and energies outlined in this book are only intended as guidelines. Every woman has her own unique experience of her cycle, and external factors can also influence how women experience their Optimum Times. This makes it important for communication to be two-way, with women giving men the information they need to adapt their approach and expectations to align with women's Optimum Times.

Why bother?

Optimum Times have an important part to play in women's everyday life, in their work, their relationships and within the family.

When women are given the environment to express themselves according to their Optimum Times, they can experience a huge drop in stress and greater feelings of fulfillment, self-confidence, well-being and happiness. They also have an enhanced capacity to achieve more in their life, to create personal success and to fulfill their goals and dreams.

"As a male professional business and life coach I can freely relate to many of the concepts and observations you make about how to make best use of the female "phases" during the course of each month. I am very fortunate to have the opportunity to work with many business women who I believe would benefit from understanding this powerful approach rather than fighting with it..." Ian Dickson, Master coach, UK, www.action-coaching.co.uk.

At work, women have the capacity to exceed productivity and efficiency, create happy and motivated teams, and generate groundbreaking solutions and revolutionary ideas, as well as having the potential to make companies and organizations leaders in their market areas.

Whether you apply your knowledge of Optimum Times at work or to personal relationships, you will need to be flexible and keep in mind the idea of the '4 in 1' woman.

Making the effort to understand women's different Optimum Times brings great relationship rewards, and if you get it wrong this month, you always have a second chance next month!

Afterword

Riding the Optimized Wave

By working on the appropriate task within our Optimum Times we ride a **wave of excellence**, working at our highest level of ability and performance throughout the whole month.

For example, where possible, I rode my skill peak while producing this book.

I rode the Optimized Wave by using my *Dynamic* phase to edit and plan chapters, my *Expressive* phase to share my ideas, my *Creative* phase to write, and my *Reflective* phase to check that what I had written was in-tune with my heartfelt aim for the book.

Riding the Optimized Wave is not just for individuals. By taking our knowledge of our Optimum Times into the workplace, women working together can 'ride the wave'. With awareness of each other's cycles women have the opportunity to allocate tasks to the individual who is experiencing her Optimum Time for

"My sister and I own and run a business together. Since hearing Miranda's lecture on 'Optimum Times' we have started incorporating these concepts into our business structure. When we get together to discuss upcoming projects and even mundane chores that need to get finished, we check in on where we each are in our menstrual cycles and assign work between us accordingly. Not only does it improve our overall business efficiency, but it makes work so much more enjoyable when you get to say – 'That task doesn't resonate with where I am in my cycle, would you mind doing it instead?' How fabulous is that?!" Amy Sedgwick, Registered Occupational Therapist, Red Tent Sisters, Canada.

that particular task.

This means that instead of waiting a month for an individual's heightened ability to re-occur, a project can be constantly supported and sustained by the combined enhanced abilities of all the women within the project. They ride the wave of Optimum Time abilities.

This is good news for women because it helps them to both excel at what they are doing and to express all aspects of their cycles. It leads to feeling less stressed at work and more fulfilled by the work that they do.

This approach is also good news for companies and organizations because they directly benefit from the heightened skills, greater productivity and efficiency, and powerful insight and creativity their female staff have to offer. Also a happier and less stressed staff creates a much more productive environment.

The impact of the concept of Optimum Times and riding the Optimum Wave has the potential to affect and change many aspects of society, including women's education and training, therapy, aptitude and medical assessment, life and business coaching, as well as business expectations and work practice.

A uniquely female approach

Optimizing our lives is the start of a new way of viewing ourselves, our abilities, how we interact with the world, and how we can create the success, excellence, fulfillment and happiness we want in life. It offers us a positive and empowering image of a uniquely female approach, which when applied at an everyday level shows us its true worth both personally and commercially.

To live within our cycles takes courage. It means stepping out of the box in the way we live, work and view ourselves, but we cannot grow into our full potential if we keep ourselves contained within a linear framework. By being willing to step outside the 'norm', to change from linear to cyclic, we will begin to see the benefits in all aspects of our lives.

There will obviously be times when we will feel that our emotions, physical symptoms and mental states are too much to handle, and any thought of a positive aspect to the cycle seems like a fantasy. We all experience months like these, but our perspective will change with our phases, and we have the

"I feel more and more that it's about riding a powerful wave that moves through me - on the one hand there are things that I can do to plan ahead and be in harmony with what is to come, but there is also such a spontaneous element of surrender." Sophia, Doula and Workshop facilitator, Spain.

opportunity each month to discover and change the underlying issues behind our thoughts about our cycles. Our cycles are a part of who we are and they are there for us to return to.

Living within our cycles becomes a way of life. Every cycle offers exciting and challenging opportunities to grow and develop, to heal and to be true to ourselves, to excel and to manifest the life we desire. By working with our cycles we gain new power and choices in how our lives will unfold.

I heard a lovely comment by a man on the radio the other day. He said that his mother had been 'a woman who was like the sea; she was ever changing but always the same'. This amazing perception is sadly one few women have about themselves.

Appendix 1

Creating a detailed Cycle Dial

The Optimized Woman Daily Plan is designed as an introduction to your Optimum Times and cyclic nature. The variety of changes which can occur during the monthly cycle however is much more diverse than those covered in the plan.

Below are a series of tables outlining just a few of the changes experienced by women during their menstrual cycles. Look through these tables and tick the experiences which you encounter in your own cycle.

Obviously it's extremely time-consuming to record all these changes over a month, so choose to record those which impact on your life the most, whether you perceive them as positive or negative experiences. Focus on creating a Cycle Dial for these identified changes.

At the end of the month, review your dial and think of some positive and practical ways of applying your experiences. See if you can come up with some ways to actively support yourself in the month ahead.

You can photocopy and enlarge the blank Cycle Dial in *Appendix 2,* or there is a version to download at
www.optimizedwoman.com for personal use.

Table 1 Mental experiences

Attention to detail	Concentration level	Ease of learning new things
Ambitions	Aims	Positive / negative thinking
Chaotic/logical thought processes	Ability to plan	Ability to articulate, express ideas and communicate well
Ability to focus	Tactical thinking	Ability to cope with numerous tasks, concepts and pressures
Ability to understand complex information	Overview thinking	Ability to make the 'right' decisions / choices
Ability to day dream	Being critical	Being judgmental
Need for structure	Flexibility	Over-thinking and worry
Need for details	Need to understand	Ability to problem solve
Inspiration	Mental clarity	Ability to visualize
Need for control	Good memory recall	Ego-orientated / people centric
Need for new projects	Commitment	Need for creative projects

Being bored, needing new experiences and change	Tolerance	Patience
Ability to let go	Ability to quieten the mind and meditate	Self belief, assertiveness
Need for attention and validation	Reaction to stress	Reactions to people –sociable / antisocial

Table 2 Physical experiences

Energy levels	Need for sleep	Need for physical action
Vitality Co-ordination and spatial awareness	Stamina Flexibility	Strength Ability to slow down and relax
Need for sensual experiences	Low or high sex drive	Self pleasure
Erotic sex drive	How you move and walk	Need for physical touch and reassurance
How people react to your physical appearance	Need for physical creative activities	Changes in diet
Cravings and addictions	Physical changes, e.g. weight, fluid retention, breast shape	Pain thresholds

Changes in the senses, e.g. sight, hearing, sense of smell	Sense of personal space	Feeling hot or cold

Table 3 Emotions and feelings

Enthusiasm	Anxiety	Paranoia
Emotional security and commitment	Fear	Feeling loving, altruistic and open
Feeling you belong	Feeling successful	Feeling secure and empowered
Passion	Grief	Compassion
Empathy	Anger and aggression	Feeling victimized
Happiness	Peacefulness	Contentment
Empowerment	Optimism / pessimism	Self-confidence
Nurturing	Emotional need for change	Emotional sensitivity / dispassion
Connecting with others	Need for emotional support and reassurance	Need to let go and move on
The types of men you are attracted to.	The things you need to feel happy	Forgiveness
Enjoying giving	Enjoying being helped	Being happy to be told

		what to do
Sudden emotional changes	Experiencing well-being, completeness and happiness	Being emotionally reactive
The need to be 'right' or have your opinions validated	Needing to help others to feel self-worth	Needing others' good opinion to feel self-worth
Demanding or needy sex	Reaction to criticism	Independence / co-dependence
Loving sex, dispassionate sex		

Table 4 Spirituality and intuition

Intuition	Spirituality	Spontaneity
Inner peace	Inner knowledge	Inner confidence
Need for religious support and experience	Need for spiritual purpose for goals and life	Dreams, e.g. positive, negative, sexual, predictive, processing, spiritual.
Spiritual sexuality	Realizations	Psychic abilities
Eureka moments		

Appendix 2

Resources and reference

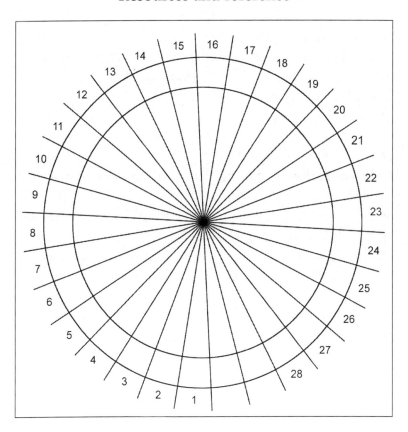

Workshops

UK

Miranda Gray is based in Hampshire, England and 'Optimized Woman' talks and workshops are run by her worldwide. Miranda also runs an online life-coaching course for women based on the menstrual cycle. For more information, visit the 'Optimized Woman' website. Her book *Red Moon - Understanding and using the*

gifts of the menstrual cycle is also available via the website.
Email: enquiries@optimizedwoman.com
Website: www.optimizedwoman.com

Spain

Sophia Style runs workshops in Spain to enable women to connect in a practical and inspirational way with the wisdom of their menstrual cycle. Based in Girona, Cataluña, Spain.
Tel: 00 34 972 77 18 51.
Email: semillas@pangea.org

Canada

Red Tent Sisters is run by **Amy Sedgwick** and **Kimberley Sedgwick**. It is a Toronto-based retail and service business dedicated to the reproductive and sexual health of women. Red Tent Sisters aims to provide a safe-haven for women to explore issues of menstruation, sexuality, childbirth, and the cyclic phases of womanhood. Their products and services emphasize a commitment to ecology, body literacy and reproductive empowerment.
Tel: 416-463-TENT (8368).
Email: info@redtentsisters.com
Website: www.redtentsisters.com

'**The Moon Goddess Series**'- yoga, mediation and the moon cycle, with **Zahra Haji**. The eight class series integrates Ten Body Kundalini yoga, offering specific yoga sets and meditations relating to the four phases. Distance education coming soon. Based in Toronto, Canada.
Tel: 416 707 6294.
Email: iam@yoga-goddess.ca
Website: www.yoga-goddess.ca

Sexual Health Access Alberta based in Calgary, facilitates access to comprehensive sexual health information, education and services. With a focus on public education and advocacy, SHAA engages the public in discussions about a broad range of issues including the menstrual suppression debate. The organization is raising questions about how the sexual health community teaches menstrual cycle awareness to inform women's reproductive health choices and support those seeking alternatives to hormonal contraception.

Tel: 403 283-8591
E-mail: info@sexualhealthaccess.org
Website: www.sexualhealthaccess.org

USA
Red Moon - Cycles of Women's Wisdom™ with **DeAnna L'am**: Make peace with your menstrual cycle. Welcome girls into womanhood with ease and authenticity. Fall in love with being a woman! Workshops, consultations, trainings worldwide.
Email: lam@sonic.net.
Website: www.deannalam.com

Further reading

The list below contains references and suggested titles to read during the different phases of the cycle.

Dynamic phase
Instant Confidence
by Paul McKenna
UK publisher: Bantam Press 2006
US publisher: Bantam Press 2006

Thresholds of the mind
by Bill Harris
USA publisher: Centerpointe Press 2002

The Cosmic Ordering Service
by Barbel Mohr
UK publisher: Mobius 2006
US publisher: Hampton Roads Publishing Company 2001

Be Your Own Life Coach: How to Take Control of Your Life and Achieve Your Wildest Dreams
by Fiona Harrold
UK publisher: Hodder Mobius 2001
US publisher: Hodder Headline2001

NLP in 21 Days: A Complete Introduction and Training Programme
by Harry Alder and Beryl Heather
UK publisher: Piatkus Books 1999

Expressive phase

How to Win Friends and Influence People
by Dale Carnegie
UK publisher: Vermilion 2007
US publisher: Vermilion 2007

Nonviolent Communication: a Language of Life
by Marshall B. Rosenberg
US publisher: Puddle Dancer Press 2003

The Wise Wound
by Penelope Shuttle and Peter Redgrove
UK publisher: Marion Boyars Publishers Ltd 2005
US publisher: Marion Boyars Publishers Ltd 2005

Creative phase
Get Everything Done and Still Have Time to Play
by Mark Forster
UK publisher: Hodder & Stoughton 2000
US publisher: McGraw-Hill 2001

The Ultimate Book of Mind Maps
by Tony Buzan
UK publisher: Harper Thorsons 2006
US publisher: Thorsons 2005

Stop Thinking, Start Living: Discover Lifelong Happiness
by Richard Carlson
UK publisher: Element 1997
US publisher: Thorsons 1997

The Sedona Method: Your Key to Lasting Happiness, Success, Peace and Emotional Well-being
by Hale Dwoskin
UK publisher: Element Books 2005
USA publisher: (with Jan Canfield) Sedona Press 2003

One Minute For Yourself: A Simple Strategy for a Better Life
by Spencer Johnson
UK publisher: HarperCollins Entertainment 2005
US publisher: HarperCollins Entertainment 2005

Reflective phase
The Secret
by Rhonda Byrne)
UK publisher: Simon & Schuster Ltd 2006
US publisher: Atria Books/Beyond Words 2006

Visual Journaling: Going Deeper Than Words
by Barbara Ganim and Susan Fox
US publisher: Quest Books, U.S. 1999

Women Who Run with the Wolves: Contacting the Power of the Wild Woman
by Clarissa Pinkola Estes
UK publisher: Rider & Co 2008
US publisher: Ballantine Books 2003

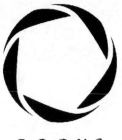

BOOKS

O is a symbol of the world, of oneness and unity. In different cultures it also means the "eye," symbolizing knowledge and insight. We aim to publish books that are accessible, constructive and that challenge accepted opinion, both that of academia and the "moral majority."

Our books are available in all good English language bookstores worldwide. If you don't see the book on the shelves ask the bookstore to order it for you, quoting the ISBN number and title. Alternatively you can order online (all major online retail sites carry our titles) or contact the distributor in the relevant country, listed on the copyright page.

See our website **www.o-books.net** for a full list of over 500 titles, growing by 100 a year.

And tune in to myspiritradio.com for our book review radio show, hosted by June-Elleni Laine, where you can listen to the authors discussing their books.

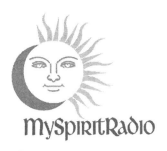

MySpiritRadio

Printed and bound by CPI Group (UK) Ltd, Croydon, CR0 4YY